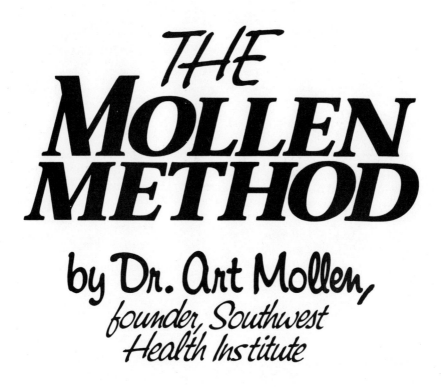

THE MOLLEN METHOD

by Dr. Art Mollen,
founder, Southwest
Health Institute

A 30-Day Program to Lifetime Health Addiction

Rodale Press, Emmaus, Pennsylvania

Book design by Anita G. Patterson

Printed in the United States of America on recycled paper containing a high percentage of de-inked fiber.

Library of Congress Cataloging-in-Publication Data

Mollen, Art.
    The Mollen method.

    Includes index.

    1. Health.   2. Exercise.   3. Nutrition.   I. Title.
RA776.M73   1986   613   85-28103
ISBN 0-87857-598-7   hardcover

2   4   6   8   10   9   7   5   3   hardcover

Notice

The information and ideas in this book are for educational purposes and must not be taken as prescriptive advice. Self-treatment can be dangerous, so consult your physician if you have a serious health problem.

CONTENTS

This book is dedicated to my children, Bradley Jason, Jenny Ann and Samantha Ann. As innocent as they are, may they learn the most important lesson of life, that of self-respect of body, mind and soul. This book is an extension of my love for them.

ACKNOWLEDGMENTS

A special acknowledgment to the Firestone family for their sagaciousness and inspiration in bringing the publication of this book to fruition, specifically Lady Julia and Lady Wray.

Gratitude is extended to Bob Barrett and Debora Tkac for their contributions.

Special thanks to my typing and research staff, Amanda Rath, Liba Lerner, Charlene Grove and Cheryl Baker, for their assistance and patience.

Thanks to all my past, present and future patients for their positive metamorphosis, both physically and emotionally. They have been and will continue to be the source of my determination to preach the message of health and fitness.

And thanks to my mother for being so proud and loving . . . it truly helps.

Chapter 1

LET'S GET MOLLENIZED!

Most people start the Mollen Method as devout skeptics. Why should the Mollen Method be any different than other fitness and weight-control programs? Is it easier? Is it more fun? What's the gimmick? Probably none of the above. But it *is* addictive.

So, what exactly is the Mollen Method, you ask? What *is* this regimen that's going to change my life around?

It's simply a diet that is easy to follow with foods that are accessible to you—but it's a diet that depends on an extra element in order to work, one that requires only ten minutes a day of your time. Ten minutes of what, you're asking? Ten minutes of moving your body parts more than you are right at this moment! Okay, call it exercise if you want to, but it will only be exercise that is fun and easy—no pain, no suffering—and it can be almost any exercise that you like. In addition to the diet and exercise, the Mollen Method will generate a positive mental attitude and a new purpose for you.

All combined, the Mollen Method offers you an improved physical, mental, emotional and spiritual being. That's a hefty load of promises, I know. And you want to know what makes me so sure that I can deliver. My confidence is based on the more than 10,000 patients I've treated at my Southwest Health Institute in Phoenix, Arizona, who have all been "Mollenized." There is nothing gimmicky, magical or even revolutionary about my program. It simply follows reasonable and sound medical guidelines and takes human nature into account.

Is your interest piqued now? Then read on. I'll give you a brief preview as to what you can expect from the 30-day Mollen plan.

The 30-Day Fat-Shaving Plan

The first week of the program will be the most difficult since you'll be exercising every day, something many of you may have never done before. Your body will probably rebel with a few minor aches and pains, suggesting the ever-common excuse of an allergic reaction to exercise.

The first week of the eating plan will be the toughest, too, but the mere motivation of starting a weight-loss program is enough to get you through. Each week the diet "guidelines" get easier.

So, what is this diet? How is it different from other diets?

The basics of the diet include salads, fruits, vegetables and fish—but in quantities larger than you've ever experienced on previous weight-loss diets. No tiny servings, one ounce of this and two ounces of that, starving you like a refugee. There are enough starving refugees in the world without adding you to the list. In fact, I never suggest eating less than 1,000 calories daily. And you can have as many as 2,000 calories! What this diet cuts out is fat—it is reduced to as low as 5 percent the first week. But this quickly increases to 10 percent, 15 percent and finally to 20 percent over the four-week period—right where you'll want to stay for a lifetime of health. See, I told you. The diet really does get easier! The motivation to keep on going will come easily as you feel the pounds melt away.

But what's the magic to the Mollen Method that will make you melt away your middle? Well, there isn't any. My diet works for a number of *logical* reasons. It's sparked by daily exercise which, studies have proven, enhances your metabolism, helping you burn calories faster and more efficiently. You'll therefore be burning more calories while you're sitting at your desk, riding in your car and even sleeping. Exercise will also tone your muscles, making you look more trim, even if weight loss isn't showing up on the scale. And, what's more, muscle requires more energy to function than fat, so you'll be burning more calories in that way, too.

In addition, you'll significantly increase your daily dose of fiber or "roughage," as your mother might have called it—fruits, vegetables, breads and other grains—which, in turn, will increase the movement of waste through your bowel. That means fat moves through you faster, too—and fewer of its calories are absorbed.

You'll also be eliminating red meat. That's right, no red meat for 30 days. Meat is naturally high in fat and since this is a *low*-fat diet and you don't want to starve (remember, I promised that you will get your fill of certain foods), you'll simply have to give it up.

I know that you're thinking that even 30 *minutes* is too long. Just the thought of giving up beef is going to give you a Big Mac attack! Believe me, the fast food industry of this country can live without you for the next 30 days. I'm not saying you must give up red meats forever, simply for the next 30 days. Take it from my patients: "It isn't hard to do at all." I tried it 12 years ago and haven't had any meat since. The good news is that you can compensate with lean fish and poultry and eat salads, fruits and vegetables to your heart's content. You can even have bread! Trust me, the diet works. Are you going to argue with success?

Ten Minutes a Day Keeps the Flab Away

The dieting you can handle, you say. But exercise? Every day? No way. Well, I'm not surprised; I hear that all the time. But not for long. My patients learn to love exercise and you will too. That's because weight loss is a great motivator. And who can balk when all I ask is ten minutes a day. (Of course, you can do more, but I'll get to that later.)

But why ten minutes? Because ten minutes is the minimal addictive dose. That's right. If you exercise ten minutes each and every day—and I mean ten honest minutes of *real* exercise—I can pretty much guarantee that by the end of the 30 days you will become addicted to exercise. You will *want* to exercise. You will want to increase your weight loss, improve your health. You'll realize exercise is not a struggle; it's a joy!

Don't try to tell me you tried it before and it didn't work. I can bet you didn't try ten minutes a day. You probably tried more. You took on too much too fast and ended up either injured or discouraged or even both. The point is you gave up. Anyone, especially someone who is overweight and out of shape, who goes out and tries to run three miles for the first time in their life is going to feel lousy doing it (if, in fact, they can do it at all). Studies have shown a very high dropout rate for previously sedentary adults who start an exercise program at 30 to 40 minutes a shot.

So, don't go the way of these folks. Start out gradually and break into it, just like you would a new pair of shoes. All it requires is commitment— every day and preferably at the same time every day. Don't make the mistake of postponing your exercise time, for you may fall into the trap encountered by so many others before you. It will cause a loosening in the link that keeps the chain around the Mollen Method. So do it every day, same time. And no excuses! Missing a day and trying to make it up the next day may work with birth control pills, but it doesn't work with the Mollen Method.

You don't even have to take your ten minutes all at one time—if in the beginning you genuinely can't handle it. I'll allow you to divide the dosage in half—five minutes in the morning and five minutes in the afternoon. If you're already a hand at exercise and ten minutes is not enough to stimulate you, then double it by doing ten minutes in the morning and ten in the afternoon. It can only improve your chances of losing weight.

Put Fun into Your Exercise

The idea is to make exercise fun. And I'm going to show you how to make it fun. I'm not going to turn you into a marathon runner. You may not choose to run at all. There's no problem with that. In fact, I'm not going to ask you to run.

You don't want to go out for a walk, either? That's fine, too. I'll give you other choices. There are loads of them. So many, in fact, that I'm going to take away your excuses for *not* exercising. There are no excuses!

So you're a business executive who travels a lot and won't go outside to exercise in Detroit in the winter when the snow is knee deep. Or in Phoenix in the summer when it's 110°F. Then don't go outside. But don't give up exercise! I will show you later just how you can handle that. Alone. In the confines of a hotel room.

You say you're a housewife and you've got kids and no free time? That's no problem either. I'll show you how to manage that time and how to work in an exercise program to go along with the diet so that you can follow the Mollen Method and feel good about yourself.

Just as some people are more or less sensitive to medications, so are some more or less sensitive to exercise. Therefore, I will show you in Chapter 4 how to individualize your program to meet your own needs.

Think Yourself Thin

Right now, though, I want you to try to visualize yourself doing exercise *every day*, just like those trim people you admire and see aerobicizing around your neighborhood. Visualize yourself getting up in the morning and gracefully going through your program—with ease. This positive mental imagery is your first step in making it really happen.

One patient of mine credited the entire success of her diet to the fact that she constantly had a mental image of herself 50 pounds thinner, just as she had been ten years before. She said her determination became relentless.

However, when she eventually got where she wanted to be she discovered it wasn't her new body she admired as much as the fortitude it took to get there. Now, she says, "I love my new physical look *and* my new mental outlook."

Pat, another patient of mine (you'll be hearing a lot from her in this book), uses positive imagery to keep herself thin. She visualizes herself at her heaviest–90 pounds heavier than she is now. She says the mere thought of how awful she looked keeps her on the Mollen Method.

"I hated the way I felt about myself so much that the people around me reacted with negative energy when I was around.

"I'll always remember myself heavier, it's so vivid in my mind. In fact, I still see myself as 'chipmunk cheeks' and 'porky.' I keep a certain image of that in my mind, just so I won't forget how good it feels to look the way I do right now."

Whether it's a nude picture of yourself pasted to the refrigerator door, a calorie chart hanging from the ceiling or a picture of someone you'd like to look like taped to your mirror, positive visualization and reinforcement can help you to stick with the program and help to get you where you want to be.

How Much Weight Can You Lose?

Now I'll answer the question that all my patients ask: "If I'm conscientious and follow all your instructions, how much weight can I expect to lose in 30 days?"

How's 20 pounds for an answer? Does that sound motivating enough? Of course you have to be a good 20 pounds or more overweight to shed all that in 30 days. In truth, though, the important thing is not how much weight you lose in 30 days, but that you continue to lose it–gradually.

What you can realistically lose in 30 days depends on a number of factors–how much weight you need to lose, how much muscle tone you started with, your metabolic rate and your ability to stick with the Mollen Method. In addition, your body composition will make a difference, and initially you may lose more inches than pounds.

Although it's possible to lose 20 pounds, an 8- to 10-pound weight loss in 30 days is by far more medically sound. And that's what I want you to aim for–steady, weekly weight loss until you shed the weight you don't want–whether it's 20 pounds or 200! On the Mollen Method the byword isn't fast weight loss, it's permanent weight loss. Remember, you didn't put weight on overnight, so don't expect to lose it that quickly either.

Call for a Shot of Mollenium

Since I cannot come into your home and observe your eating and exercise habits over the next 30 days, I'm going to trust you to follow my directions just as you are going to trust me to help you lose weight. But I don't expect miracles. *Everyone* feels a slip in willpower once in a while. And that can be fatal. But you needn't fear. I'll be there to give you a boost with a shot of "Mollenium."

So what is Mollenium? It's the 132nd element known to man. A massive dose of motivation compounded with high energy. No, it's not kryptonite, capable of felling a Superman, but it is capable of felling your most prized excuses for giving in to temptation.

If you need a dose of Mollenium, just call 1-602-BODY-4-86 to receive motivation, energy, willpower, understanding and sympathy. I will also help you to overcome excuses, enhance attitude and increase enthusiasm about life. Just pick up the phone and I will be right there to guide you through your toughest times.

"Go for It"

I'm often asked where I get the energy to do all the things I accomplish daily. I simply reply "from within." I have a positive mental attitude about

---

A PERSONAL DOSE OF MOLLENIUM

For those of you who like to use mnemonics to remember your daily commitments, the following is for you: "I AM SEXY"

I—is for I can do it.
A—is for alcohol—reduce it.
M—is for mental attitude—make sure it's positive.
S—is for smoking—stop.
E—is for eating—control it.
X—is for exercise—do it daily.
Y—is for yes . . . I can make my goal come true.

This book contains little hints that I've learned about motivating people to exercise. Since I've learned the rules by which the game of health and fitness is played, I also realize there are no shortcuts.

If you are afraid of being motivated and changing your lifestyle, then put this book down immediately and go on your way, for the surgeon general of this book has warned, "Exercise may be beneficial to your health."

myself and the world around me. It allows me to deal positively with the people I meet each day.

In fact, at least once a week a negative and unhappy person walks into my office expressing skepticism about me and the Mollen Method but leaves with a positive, confident feeling about the changes soon to be experienced.

My good friend and patient Tex Earnhardt is an example of what positive energy can do for you. Tex, one of the largest automobile dealers in America, came to me more than ten years ago because of stress and high blood pressure. Says Tex today, "I've never felt better than I do right now. The exercise and diet have given me more energy, more stamina and the most positive mental attitude that a man could have. If I don't run six miles every day, I just don't feel right. I'd hate to say that I can't live without exercise, but it is the most important part of my day."

Tex exemplifies positive energy. Perhaps it's a cliché, but he often refers to his attitude about life as a "constant high."

You, too, can be like Tex and be high on life. All you need to do is learn how to achieve it. It doesn't come from financial security, a pretty face or material possessions. It comes from good health and mental well-being. And the way you get it all starts with diet and exercise.

So, let's make the commitment for the next 30 days. By month's end, I'm certain you'll feel so good about yourself you'll want to continue the Mollen Method forever. Thirty days, ten minutes a day—it's the minimal addictive dose that I can prescribe for you.

The time to get started is now. Not tomorrow, not Monday, not the Monday after the next holiday. If at the end of the 30 days, you don't like the way you feel or haven't developed more self-confidence, then simply burn this book, or give it to someone you don't like. Of course, I don't expect this to happen. In fact, I think you'll experience the antithesis and find yourself addicted to a daily dose of Mollenium.

Chapter 2
TAKE A LOOK AT YOURSELF

I'm not a faith healer, I'm not a movie star and I'm not a professional athlete. I'm a doctor. I keep myself in shape by exercising and eating right. I do it because I want to stay healthy, and also because it makes me feel good about myself.

All day long I see patients who are overweight and out of shape and can't get motivated to do something about it. They stand in front of the mirror looking at their bulges and flab and feel bad about themselves. They sometimes won't put on a bathing suit, or even look for a job. They're defeated because of their physical appearance and they're depressed, too.

I help these patients, and I can help you, too. All you have to do is change your *attitude*, and everything else will change with it. That's part of the Mollen Method: The positive attitude that I instill in my patients helps them change the self-defeating behaviors that have them fighting their weight.

Here's where we start: Think for a moment about what is your most valuable possession. If you're like most of my patients when I ask that question, you immediately name something material like a car, a house or an art object.

"No," I tell them. "Your most valuable possession in life is your physical being."

Once I say that, they usually agree. But you'd be surprised how few people actually begin by thinking of themselves as their most prized possession.

If you agree that your physical being is your most valuable possession, then why do you treat it the way you do?

Think about it right now and focus for a minute on one of your prized possessions: the car, the house, an art object, almost anything. I'll bet you treat it better than you treat your physical being. If you picked your car, you probably clean it, tune it, and take care of it. If you picked the art object, you protect it from excessive moisture and from theft.

But what do you do for your physical being—your most valuable possession? You misuse it by overeating, not getting enough exercise, and abusing alcohol.

Worst of all, when we do these things, we hate ourselves. It's a downward spiral; we're fat and flabby, so we feel depressed. Because we're depressed, we eat and drink some more.

That doesn't have to happen. You are never too old, too fat or too out of shape to make a big improvement in your physical being. There is no age limit on getting in shape—anyone can do it. How? By making up your mind to do it. By changing your attitude. It starts with the commitment that you are going to treat your physical being as your most valuable possession. Doing this will change your life!

That may sound corny, but think about it. You owe the material things you always thought of as your most valuable possessions to your ability to make money. And your ability to make money depends on the condition of your physical being—your health and your appearance.

Most people start their day at a 6 on a scale of 1 to 10. They drink coffee to get going and hope to begin feeling like an 8, but by the end of the day with everybody slam-dunking them and wearing them down, down, down, they finish tired and worn out, often finishing at −1 and reaching up to touch bottom.

But people who have control of their lives, who have improved the quality of their lives with diet and exercise, start the day beyond a 10. They start somewhere around 13, just because they are feeling so good about themselves. They go through the day and get worn down, but they finish the day feeling like a 7 and have energy left over to go out in the evening.

This is what I tell my patients. Make the commitment, change your negatives to positives and you, too, will be starting your day on a high instead of a low. You must feel good about yourself *within* before you can expect to notice the changes *without*. Diet and exercise go hand in hand with feeling good about yourself.

So take a look at yourself. Get control of your feelings and turn off all those negatives. As far as I'm concerned, no one is beyond hope as long as they go after what they want with a positive attitude.

Need a little inspiration? Then listen to what the right spirit did for some of my patients.

Hope for the Hopeless

When Karen first came to see me, she was miserable. At age 38, she was 30 pounds overweight and in a rocky marriage. Once the high school beauty queen, now she admitted to not even liking herself very much.

I made Karen commit herself to valuing her physical being above all else. Together, we seized control of her life. She lost 30 pounds and looked great. Her relationship with her husband improved. Her eyes sparkled. Her hair gleamed and her skin tone improved. Even her clothing had changed. Her tentlike dresses were gone, replaced by clothing that revealed her new shape. Now I could see the beauty queen that she'd remembered.

Karen was excited about going back East on a business trip with her husband—the first time she'd ever been invited to go with him. It was a brand-new Karen who said to me:

"I think he just wants to show me off."

I see so many young girls come into my office with bodies that look 20 years older than their faces. But when they make the commitment to change their attitude about themselves, the physical changes come easily.

Bonnie is my best example. When Bonnie was 20 years old, she was 35 pounds overweight. She had a lovely face, but because she was overweight she didn't date very often and didn't like the men she did date. She was depressed because her more attractive friends seemed to be getting all the great guys.

Within months after coming to see me, she had lost the excess weight. She made a tentative commitment that became stronger and stronger as she started to see the payoff. She was finally meeting men she liked. The last time I saw her was at her wedding. She was a very beautiful bride.

I even had one patient who made a dream career change. After adopting the Mollen Method and losing weight, she changed careers from secretary to model.

Robert was an executive at a copper company here in Arizona. He was under a great deal of stress in his job, and he was overweight. Although Robert knew he was in line for a promotion, he wasn't sure he would get it. Worse, he was afraid if he did get it, the additional stress would kill him.

For Robert, the Mollen Method paid off quickly. Within two months he noticed increased energy at work. That meant he could do more work with less stress, even though his job hadn't changed. Robert was handling his stress better. The quality of his life had improved and so had his attitude. Robert is now president of the company.

Jerry was a mechanic. He didn't have a weight problem, but he did have an attitude problem. He also had high blood pressure. He was too uptight, snapping constantly at his customers and driving them away. Although he was only 20, Jerry knew if he didn't make some changes in his life, he'd lose his business. The Mollen Method gave Jerry control. He was able to reduce his stress, lower his blood pressure and increase his tolerance.

Then there's Susan. When Susan first came to see me, she was 33 and weighed 280 pounds. "Last New Year's I decided I had to do something about my weight once and for all. I needed to do something *serious*. I'd tried Weight Watchers and just about everything else with little success. So I decided to try again. I had to; at that time I weighed 320 pounds.

"I went on a diet, lost 40 pounds and then I stopped. About two months later I found myself going back and doing the same old things. I got scared. I thought, 'It's going to be like every other time, the same thing is going to happen.'

"The thing is, all my life I've been able to put on 30 to 40 pounds and then take it off. But I couldn't get below that."

That first day she walked into my office and simply said "Help me."

Three months and 50 pounds later she said to me: "I'll never forget what you said: 'It's not going to matter that you're going to lose the weight. What's going to matter is that you're going to feel better about yourself than you ever have in your life.' Having tried the Stillman Diet, the Atkins Diet, TOPS, Overeaters Anonymous and diets from newspapers and magazines, I didn't think this would work either, but I had to try," said Susan.

After six months she had lost 95 pounds. "I'd wanted to make it 100 pounds before I went home for a visit at Christmas," said Susan, "but I just missed. Anyway, I told my parents that I'd lost some weight and my dad just laughed over the phone. When I got off the plane my dad didn't recognize me at first. Then his mouth fell open!

"I was 95 pounds lighter, I'd changed my hairstyle and gotten contacts, my skin had cleared up and I was dressed differently. The family didn't believe it and my grandmother thought I was one of my younger sisters at first. It was great."

Susan's story is one of many that prove diet and exercise can change everything. Once you make the commitment, it isn't difficult. The Mollen Method only takes 30 days. That's one month—which can change your life forever.

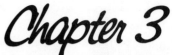

Chapter 3

HERE'S TO YOUR HEALTH

When people come to me to discuss their weight problem, they talk about the obvious difficulties—lack of energy, embarrassment about their looks, lack of attention from friends or the opposite sex. If their weight is excessive, they might talk about how bad they feel when they have to squeeze into a theater seat, or how narrow the booths are in restaurants, or how difficult it is to get clothing that looks good on them.

Few, if any, realize—or at least like to think about—the medical dangers of being overweight.

The most obvious danger, of course, is heart disease. A fat body has to work a lot harder to do the same amount of work as a thin body. And that puts excess stress on the heart. Imagine putting a 50-pound sack on your back and attempting to climb a three-story walkup. You know the going would be a lot easier without the sack.

Well, 50 pounds of excess fat is not a whole lot different. For example, depending upon physical condition, the average person's heart beats 72 to 78 times per minute. A walk up the stairs would make the number of beats go up to about 120 a minute. But add a 50-pound sack, and the average number of beats will go up to 160 per minute on that walk up those stairs. Of course, the numbers will vary from person to person but the result is the same—you're going to put more stress on the heart. Get rid of the 50-pound sack—your excess weight—and your heart will have it much easier.

Overweight also jeopardizes the heart in another way. It almost always leads to an increased amount of cholesterol in your blood (from simply eating too much of it), which eventually leads to a buildup of cholesterol and fats in the major coronary arteries of your heart. Before you know it—heart attack.

Heard it all before? Too bad. You're going to hear more.

Being overweight can also lead to diabetes, one of the major contributors to poor health. Diabetes means the pancreas is unable to furnish the proper amount of insulin necessary to regulate the body's blood sugar level. Severe cases can result in coma or even death.

Diabetes also promotes the deposit of cholesterol in your arteries and the growth of bacteria in parts of your body, which can lead to other diseases. In fact, it's more difficult for a diabetic to heal from something as simple as a cut because the bacteria thrive on a high blood sugar level.

And don't think that because no one in your family has ever had diabetes (after all, it is an "inherited" disease) you're off the hook. Not so. Native Americans—American Indians who have no history of the disease—are beginning to come down with it. Why? Because unlike their ancestors, many of them are overweight. Diabetes is becoming a problem because of their *lifestyle*.

High blood pressure or hypertension, known as the "silent killer," is another backlash of overweight. One of the reasons it is so dangerous is that so many people don't know they have it. The initial symptoms—headache, dizziness or blacking out—often lead people to the doctor seeking a diagnosis because they expect something else. If you're overweight by 20 or more pounds, you are at a significantly higher risk of developing hypertension in the future. It's wise to have your blood pressure checked.

Another serious consequence of overweight can be cancer. Studies have suggested that obese people may be more at risk for developing cancer than people of normal weight. In addition, studies have suggested that people who eat high-fat diets have an increased risk of developing cancer, especially of the bowel. Therefore, the American Cancer Society has recommended that people eat a low-fat, high-fiber diet (just like the Mollen Method) to lower their risk of developing the disease.

Arthritis is another problem for the overweight because of all the excess stress that extra weight puts on the joints. The Arthritis Foundation has suggested that arthritics control their weight in an effort to avoid progressive joint deterioration.

And the list goes on.

Sorry for the lecture. It's just that I can't stress strongly enough that overweight is much more than a cosmetic problem. And while a great-looking body is a great goal, great health is an even better one.

SMOKING? IT'S TIME TO QUIT

You say you've tried and just can't? Consider these facts. They may encourage you to give it another try:

- Smoking one pack of cigarettes a day is equal to carrying around an additional 80 pounds of weight in terms of the stress it puts on the heart.
- Smokers carry a 70 percent greater risk of developing heart disease than nonsmokers.
- Eighty-five percent of lung cancer deaths could be avoided if people didn't smoke.
- Lung cancer is now killing more women than breast cancer.
- Smokers are more susceptible to the flu than nonsmokers. Also, their bout with the flu is more severe and recovery time is slower.
- Smokers have more ulcers and gastrointestinal problems than nonsmokers.

- An estimated 250,000 Americans will die this year as a result of smoking.

It doesn't matter whether you've been smoking for 4 years or 40 years. You can still reap benefits if you stop. For instance, within one year after you quit, your chances of developing heart disease will be reduced considerably. Within ten years, the ex-smoker's risk of heart disease is the same as the person who never smoked.

Take a little inspiration from Grant Goodeve, the handsome and charming television actor. He decided to quit his pack-a-day habit after visiting my Phoenix health institute. Six months later Grant told me, "I feel better than I have in a long time. I have more energy, less fatigue, and I can breathe better since I quit."

Why don't you follow Grant's example and quit smoking today.

In Harm's Weigh? ·

Now that you know what sorts of risks you're taking if you are overweight, the big question arises: How can you tell if you are overweight? At what point do you stop being just a bit overweight and have to start seriously thinking of getting rid of that extra weight for your health's sake?

I consider people seriously overweight when they're 20 pounds or more over their ideal weight. According to the scientific community, 20 pounds is where overweight ends and obesity begins. And some 36 million Americans past age 20 fit into that category!

I don't think people have to be perfect or fanatical about their weight. But anyone carrying an extra 20 or more pounds must make a decision to do something about it or possibly face some serious consequences.

How do you know what your weight should be? You could check a weight chart. There certainly are enough of them around. Most doctors as well as insurance companies have them. Of course, this requires a bit of honesty. If you are average in size, then look at the weight for an average build. Don't decide you have a large frame just because your current weight is right for that size. In fact, some people have been known to grow an inch or two while looking at these charts!

One of the best, and easiest, ways to tell if you're overweight is to simply stand in front of a mirror—without holding in your stomach. Relax. If you can "pinch more than an inch" of flab around your waist, it's time to do something about it. Simply by looking at your image and being completely honest with yourself, you will know if you need to lose weight or not. Or you may decide that you're not overweight, just soft and out of shape. If that's the case you should still do something about it. Being "overfat" is also bad for your health. What you need to do is exchange some of the flab for muscle (you'll learn how to do this in the next chapter).

The most *accurate* way to determine if you are overweight is through an underwater submersion test. This test can determine exactly how much body fat you are carrying around. It's the method I use at my clinic. Perhaps a doctor or a clinic in your area has a testing tank.

If not, I suggest you simply allow your mirror to be your guide. But, be *honest.* Do you really like what you see? As you progress on the Mollen Method, you'll discover how unimportant the scale can be. The mirror will be the real judge of your overall improvement in the early stages. And the way you feel will be the all-important factor in the later stages—and in all the stages of your life to come.

Your Number 1 Goal: Improved Health

The Mollen Method is much more than a weight loss program. It is a program of better health. So it doesn't matter if you weigh too much, weigh too little or even if your weight is just right. *Everyone* can benefit from the Mollen Method.

Not everyone who comes to see me is looking for a weight loss program. People see me for a variety of ills—from hemorrhoids to heart disease. But for just about everyone I have one prescription—diet and exercise. Not only does it help prevent disease, but it helps people regain the health they've lost through sickness and disease. It's proven better than any pill I can recommend. In fact, handing out medication is something I try to avoid at my institute.

YOU'LL GET THAT HEALTHY FEELING

Some diet methods help you lose weight, but they wear you out and tear you down in the process. The Mollen Method, however, is a health *builder.* In addition to weight loss, this diet program can:

- Lower blood pressure
- Lower pulse rate
- Lower cholesterol levels
- Lower triglyceride levels
- Reduce risk of bowel disease
- Improve joint mobility
- Increase flexibility
- Improve muscle tone
- Improve muscle strength
- Improve complexion
- Improve self-confidence
- Improve mental attitude
- Control blood sugar levels
- Improve stress control
- Improve sleeping patterns
- Reduce nervousness
- Improve circulation

I believe our society is far too drug oriented. You get a headache, you run to the medicine cabinet and take some aspirin. As children, we got sick, were taken to the doctor and given medicine that made us feel better. Now we do the same for our own children. We were conditioned that way. It's no wonder we look for a pill as an instant cure to a problem!

In my practice, I've found that diet and exercise, individually tailored to a person, can successfully treat many conditions that other physicians are treating with medications. I've also found that diet and exercise can actually eliminate the need for surgery, costly drugs and excessive medical attention for some people. In short, the Mollen Method is therapeutic *and* preventive.

Substitute the Mollen Method for Medicine

The simple prescription of diet and exercise makes my patients feel better, reduces their symptoms and minimizes or eliminates their medication.

I realize this is a powerful statement, so before I continue, let me tell you about Mildred. When she came to see me late in 1982, Mildred was 60 years old, weighed 160 pounds and had a resting pulse rate of 84 (it should have been closer to 70). She was also taking a lot of medications—13 in all—as a result of a heart attack four years earlier.

Here's what a brand-new Mildred has to say about herself:

"I had gained a lot of weight and I was taking all this medication. I felt so exhausted all the time.

"On the Mollen Method I lost 30 pounds in eight weeks. I'm now off all medication except for one. I didn't get off all that medicine at once, though. It was gradual. In fact, I'm even off nitroglycerin, and every other doctor told me I'd never be able to stop taking it. I haven't had any problems since stopping the medication.

"The big difference in my life now is that because I exercise I've got more energy; I'm not tired all the time like I used to be. It used to be a chore to do anything. The exercising was difficult at first—my legs used to get so tired; however, I just pushed myself. If I don't exercise every day I'm done for, so I almost never miss. I know it's something I have to do; it's for my health. If I want to feel better, I have to exercise.

"I just feel so good. A couple of years ago I couldn't do anything but take medicine. Today I'm running races. It's exciting."

Before you say, "Yes, but Mildred is the exception," I want you to know that Mildred is *not* the exception. I have plenty of patients just like her.

Now, I'm not recommending that you adopt the Mollen Method and stop taking your medication. But I am suggesting that with careful supervision by your physician, adopting the Mollen Method could help you *control* your condition. The amount of medication you take is for you and your physician to determine, so be sure to consult with him or her before discontinuing any medication. And keep in mind that Mildred didn't stop 12 of her 13 medications all at once. It was a slow and gradual reduction.

Whether the Mollen Method wil help *you* depends upon your condition, the medication you are taking and your commitment to the program.

Now, let's take a look at some other special conditions that the Mollen Method may help. This listing is by no means complete, so if your problem isn't here, there is still a chance that the Mollen Method can make a difference—the difference—in the quality of your life. Talk it over with your doctor.

Help for Arthritics

Have you ever awakened in the morning with pain and stiffness in your joints? Once you started moving around, however, you were fine. Millions of Americans suffering from arthritis wake up feeling this way, but they get progressively worse during the day and receive only moderate relief from medication.

Arthritis is the loss of movement in a joint due to a calcification in that particular joint space. Osteoarthritis is most common in the elderly. Rheumatoid arthritis usually occurs earlier in life. Gout, another form of arthritis, is due to more of a metabolic process in which uric acid accumulates in the joints. Gout may occur at any time.

Rheumatoid arthritis and osteoarthritis cannot be cured. They can only be treated and partially relieved.

Treatment of arthritis over the years has varied. However, aspirin remains the treatment of choice. Steroids will relieve the arthritis but not without serious consequences when taken over a long term.

Does that mean that if you have arthritis all you can do is take aspirin until it is so bad you have to begin steroids?

Not at all. The Mollen Method can help.

I have treated my arthritic patients with exercise and diet. I have found that the diet that works quite effectively consists of ample amounts of salads, fruits and vegetables with occasional juice fasting. I suggest a juice fast (8 to 10 glasses a day of vegetable juices only), for 24 hours once a week. For those who are more severely affected, I suggest a 48-hour juice fast weekly. Here are my guidelines for the antiarthritic juice fast:

• Vegetable juices, including carrot, cabbage, celery and tomato
• No canned juices; make your own (a home juicer is a good investment)
• Avoid fruit juices such as orange, apple and pineapple
• 24 hours once a week for mild cases
• 48 hours once a week for moderate to severe cases

Why a juice fast? The juice fast has an anti-inflammatory effect on the body. It puts the body through a catharsis that reduces joint inflammation and improves joint mobility.

None of this diet is revolutionary; it's nothing for which I can lay claim. Leading nutritionists have suggested this type of diet in the treatment of arthritis for years. (Of course, you should consult your doctor before undertaking any type of fast.) By adding exercise to the prescription, you will enhance joint movement even more. Studies have suggested that exercise increases the flow and oxygenation of the blood going to the joints, helping them to move better.

Other studies have suggested that exercise increases endorphins in the brain. Endorphins are morphinelike chemicals that relieve pain. An increase in endorphins raises the pain threshold and allows arthritics to tolerate pain better. Some of the studies suggest that this is why arthritics feel better when they exercise.

More than 75 percent of my patients with arthritis have claimed an improvement after following the Mollen Method for just 30 days. In addition to the juice fast, my arthritic patients follow the regular Mollen Method low-fat diet for maximum relief. The longer you stay with the diet the greater the improvements and benefits.

Exercise and Arthritis

How should someone with arthritis exercise?

It depends on the person and the severity of the condition. Aerobic exercise is, of course, the most beneficial.

If an arthritic can walk, that is my first suggestion for exercise. My second suggestion is stationary bicycling. The outdoor bicycle requires balance and for elderly people it may be risky. Swimming is also an excellent exercise for arthritics, as it facilitates joint movement and minimizes stress on muscles and joints.

One last exercise for arthritics is jogging. I know that may shock many of you. However, there is no contraindication to a jogging program for arthritics.

Exercise will not reverse or cure arthritis but exercise will help to relieve it. In addition, it may cause the disease to go into a remission.

Benefits for Wheelchair Patients

Perhaps you're saying that's fine for those fortunate enough to be able to get up and walk, but what if the arthritis is worse? What if the arthritic is so severely crippled he or she is confined to a wheelchair and unable to walk for exercise?

Arthritics who are unable to walk (or anyone confined to a wheelchair) should use their upper body as much as possible. Upper body exercises burn up a lot of calories because the upper body muscles are not as efficient as those in the legs. Upper body muscles require more energy to perform a similar task done more easily by your legs.

I suggest that wheelchair arthritics buy a stationary bicycle, place it on a table and pedal it with their arms. Do this initially for five minutes, slowly building up to at least ten minutes daily. Five minutes of bicyling with the arms at a reasonable speed would be the equivalent of a mile of walking. Do whatever amount at whatever intensity you can tolerate.

Does it work? Can those in a wheelchair pedal a stationary bicycle by hand and improve their arthritis?

Yes, it happens. And it helped Glen. Glen came to me confined to a wheelchair. As a child, Glen had contracted polio and subsequently developed arthritis in almost every joint. He had a fused spine, as well as fused ankles and a fused right hip due to the arthritis. He was also experiencing rapid heartbeats and was on a variety of medications when he came to my office.

This is what Glen had to say about the Mollen Method:

"I had severe arthritis for about 13 years and had been on heavy dosages of heart medications. There had been no improvement and my arthritis was getting worse.

"I had tried everything from cortisone to acupuncture before the Mollen Method. My last doctor said to go home and learn to live with the pain.

"All the doctors in the past had told me over and over and over: 'No exercise.' They said there was deterioration of the joints and exercise would put wear and tear on the joints. So I eliminated any exercise I was then capable of doing. I practically lost all the strength in my arms.

"I told Dr. Mollen I'd give his program 30 days. Not 31, just 30. He said if there was no improvement, then there would be no charge, either.

"By the time he took me off the last heart medication, I was up to almost 20 miles a day pedaling that bicycle. Now that's a long way with just your arms. I can reach my head now and not feel any pain. Can you imagine how wonderful it is to be able to comb your own hair? I would have to say that I haven't felt as good in 20 or 25 years.

"I have two recommendations for handicapped people," says Glen. "Do your exercises and keep your weight down. You see too many people in wheelchairs like me who are really obese.

"Now, I'm not going to say I'm cured of arthritis; I'm not. But the thing is to get relief, to control it."

I asked Glen what was the most important change that took place in his life. His answer: "A better mental attitude."

A Lower Risk of Heart Disease

When patients visit my institute, I evaluate their heart attack risk and then reevaluate them again after their first 30 days on the Mollen Method. In *all* cases, their risk goes down significantly.

Why? Because studies have proven that a lifestyle that includes a diet low in fat, a daily exercise routine, no smoking and moderate alcohol—the Mollen Method—contributes significantly in reducing the chance of developing heart disease, America's number-one killer.

MOLLEN HEART DISEASE RISK INDEX

The following is a simple test which may indicate your risk for developing heart disease some time in the future. Count the number of points that accumulate by answering the following questions:

1. *If your age is below 30 add 1*
   If your age is between 30 and 40 add 2
   If your age is between 41 and 50 add 3
   If your age is between 51 and 60 add 5
   If your age is above 60 add 7

   _____

2. *If you have no known family history of heart disease add 0*
   If one or more relatives have had heart disease below age 60 add 2

   _____

3. *If you are up to 20 pounds overweight add 1*
   If you are 20 to 50 pounds overweight add 2
   If you are 50 or more pounds overweight add 3

   _____

4. *If you smoke a cigar and/or pipe add 1*
   If you smoke less than 1 pack of cigarettes daily add 2
   If you smoke 1 pack of cigarettes daily add 4
   If you smoke more than 1 pack of cigarettes daily add 6

   _____

5. *If you exercise daily add 1*
   If you exercise moderately add 3
   If your only exercise is occupation related add 6

   _____

6. *If your most recent blood cholesterol level was between 150 and 180 add 1*
   If your most recent blood cholesterol level was between 180 and 220 add 2
   If your most recent blood cholesterol level was 220 or above add 3

   _____

Because my diet is low in fat (only 5 percent the first week), LDL (low-density lipoprotein) cholesterol—the type that's a menace to the heart—naturally falls. And it is the deposit of cholesterol plaque inside the walls of the arteries that leads to atherosclerosis. A low-fat diet also brings down triglyceride levels, one of the other major fats in the blood.

But a good diet can't take all the credit. Exercise is just as important. Some studies suggest that exercise can actually clean out the deposits of cholesterol from the artery walls. Others claim that the arteries aren't

7. *If your systolic blood pressure (upper reading) was 100 to 120 add 2*
    If your systolic blood pressure was 120 to 140 add 3
    If your systolic blood pressure was 140 to 160 add 4
    If your systolic blood pressure was 160 to 180 add 6
    If your systolic blood pressure was 180 or above add 8

    _____

Total Points _____

If your accumulation of points is:

1 to 13
Your risk for developing heart disease is below average

14 to 21
Your risk for developing heart disease is average

22 to 30
Your risk for developing heart disease is above average

30 or above
Your risk for developing heart disease is high

The Mollen Heart Disease Risk Index is designed to make you aware of the shape you are in and your potential for developing heart disease in the future. It should motivate you to change your lifestyle—follow a low-fat diet, stop smoking and start exercising!

cleaned at all but that exercise increases the size of the arteries, thereby enhancing the blood flow through them. It doesn't matter which school of thought you believe, the end result is the same: Exercise is a cholesterol fighter.

In addition, HDL (high-density lipoprotein) cholesterol—the so-called "good-guy cholesterol" that actually fights plaque buildup—is increased with exercise.

There's no doubt about it. The Mollen Method fights fat!

So why don't you take the Mollen Heart Disease Risk Index. Then repeat the test after 30 days on the Mollen Method. I'm sure you'll find the risk has been lowered.

Help for Heart Attack Victims

The Mollen Method is also an ideal program for anyone who already has heart-related problems. The same principles of low fat and exercise that help guard against getting heart disease can protect those who've had a heart attack from getting another. In addition, that feel-good-about-yourself feeling that Glen and so many of my other patients describe helps in reducing stress, which is so important to a heart attack victim.

One of my most convincing stories is that of Del Himelstein, my friend and attorney, who had a heart attack at the age of 42. After one year of following the Mollen Method, he ran the Fiesta Bowl Marathon—26 miles, 385 yards. Or perhaps the story of Edna, another heart attack victim, will impress you more. When Edna first came to my office she was jogging one mile a day. She had visited another doctor who suggested she stop running. He also increased her heart medication.

I *increased* Edna's running mileage and *decreased* her heart medication. In 1983, Edna, at age 65, broke the world's record in the marathon for women her age.

Most cardiac specialists suggest that the sooner heart attack patients can be back on their feet, the better off they are. An intensive exercise program, beginning just three months after the heart attack, can significantly reduce the chances of a recurrence. One noted Canadian doctor, Terry Cavanaugh, M.D., has for more than ten years been encouraging heart patients to exercise. In fact, in 1973—to the chagrin of many of his medical peers—seven ran and finished the Boston Marathon!

There's enough scientific evidence to convince me that some day exercise will become a major treatment for post-heart attack victims. One study divided 315 heart attack patients into two groups—a control group that didn't exercise and a group that underwent exercise training. After a four-year period, they found 20 percent fewer deaths in the people who exercised. Today there are more than a hundred cardiac rehabilitation programs in the United States that include exercise programs. That's a really encouraging sign.

Here are my guidelines to cardiac rehabilitation:

• Consult with your physician as to any physical limitation you may have as a result of your condition.

- Start exercise four to six weeks after a heart attack or bypass surgery.
- Exercise under medical supervision for the first three months after a heart attack.
- Progress at your own speed and intensity of exercise.
- Do not allow your pulse rate to get above 70 percent of maximum heart rate. (See page 48 to find out how to measure it.)
- Always try to exercise with a companion.
- Take nitroglycerin along during unsupervised exercise sessions.
- Follow the 5 percent low-fat diet guidelines as long as possible. This will help to lower cholesterol and triglyceride levels significantly.
- Increase the amount and intensity of exercise as much as can be safely tolerated.

Certain cardiac conditions may not tolerate exercise so be sure to check with your physician before starting an exercise program. Walking, jogging and bicycling are appropriate exercises for post-coronary patients.

Bring High Blood Pressure Down

As you probably know, high blood pressure is one of the major risk factors for heart disease. An estimated 23 million Americans have high blood pressure; one-third of them don't know it. If you took only ten minutes out of your day to combat high blood pressure with exercise, you would be taking huge strides toward preventing heart disease.

In fact, high blood pressure is a common ailment among the patients who visit my institute, and my success rate in bringing that pressure down is 100 percent—*if* they follow the diet and exercise program properly.

One example is Charles. Charles first came to see me when I was a physician with the U.S. Air Force. He was a 5'8" staff sergeant weighing 190 pounds who had high blood pressure and was controlling it with medication. He only laughed at me when I told him he could get off the medication and control his blood pressure with exercise and diet. It was four years later when he came into my civilian office with his blood pressure still high.

"I'm fed up with all this medication," said Charles. "I'm willing to try anything."

"Even exercise?" I asked.

"Even exercise," Charles vowed.

I put Charles on the Mollen Method and today he weighs 160 pounds and his blood pressure is a steady, safe 110/70. He's running two to three miles a day. In fact, he was recently back in my office talking about his strategy for running his first marathon.

(Continued on page 33)

SOURCES OF POTASSIUM

There's no need to worry about getting a healthy allotment of potassium (the RDA is 2,500 milligrams) on the Mollen Method. Below are some of the foods you will find on the diet that are a high source of the mineral.

Food	Portion	Potassium (in mg)	% of RDA
Potatoes, baked	1 medium	844	34
Soybeans, roasted & toasted kernels	¼ cup	834	33
Carrot juice	1 cup	720	29
Beet greens, cooked	½ cup	654	26
Avocados	½ medium	602	24
Blackstrap molasses	1 tablespoon	585	23
Watermelons	1/16 medium	560	22
Yogurt, plain, low-fat	1 cup	531	21
Sardines, Atlantic, drained solids	3 ounces	501	20
Flounder	3 ounces	498	20
Soybeans, cooked	½ cup	486	19
Lima beans	½ cup	485	19
Swiss chard, cooked	½ cup, chopped	483	19
Sunflower seeds, dry roasted	¼ cup	482	19
Yams	½ cup, cubed	455	18
Bananas	1 medium	451	18
Acorn squashes	½ cup, cubed	446	18
Honeydew melons	⅛ medium	437.5	17
Casaba melons	⅛ medium	430	17
Amaranth, cooked	½ cup	423	17
Spinach, cooked	½ cup	419	17
Cantaloupe melons	¼ medium	412.5	16
Milk, skim	1 cup	406	16
Pomegranates	1 medium	399	16
Sweet potatoes, baked	1 medium	397	16
Navy beans	½ cup	395	16
Papayas	½ medium	390	16
Chicory greens, raw	½ cup, chopped	378	15
Salmon, fillet, fresh	3 ounces	378	15
Great Northern beans	½ cup	374.5	15
Salmon, Sockeye, drained solids	3 ounces	363.4	14

Food	Portion	Potassium (in mg)	% of RDA
Plantains	½ cup, sliced	358	14
Cod	3 ounces	345	14
Cowpeas (black-eyed peas)	½ cup	344	14
Plums	3 medium	339	14
Grape juice	1 cup	334	13
Pineapple juice	1 cup	334	13
Currants	¼ cup	321	13
Bamboo shoots, cooked	½ cup, sliced	320	13
Artichokes	1 medium	316	13
Chinese cabbage (bok choi), cooked	½ cup, shredded	315	13
Kidney beans	½ cup	314.5	13
Apricots, fresh	3 medium	313	12
Prunes	5 medium	313	12
Haddock	3 ounces	297	12
Butternut squashes	½ cup, cubed	290	12
Dates	¼ cup, chopped	290	12
Nectarines	1 medium	288	11
Parsnips, cooked	½ cup, sliced	287	11
Pumpkins	½ cup, mashed	281	11
Asparagus	½ cup	279	11
Kohlrabi, cooked	½ cup, sliced	279	11
Mushrooms, cooked	½ cup, cut into pieces	277	11
Persimmons	1 medium	270	11
Beets	½ cup, sliced	266	11
Celery, cooked	½ cup, diced	266	11
Turkey, white meat	3 ounces	259	10
Okra	½ cup, sliced	257	10
Guavas	1 medium	256	10
Tomatoes, red, raw	1 medium	254	10
Kiwi fruits	1 medium	252	10
Tomatoes, green, raw	1 medium	251	10

GET YOUR CALCIUM QUOTA

Some experts in high blood pressure believe by getting 1,000 milligrams of calcium a day you can reduce the likelihood of developing the disease from 20 percent to 1 percent. But you needn't depend on high-fat dairy products, such as whole milk and cheese, to get it. Below are some foods permitted on the Mollen Method that are low in fat and provide at least 1 percent of the Recommended Dietary Allowance—800 milligrams—of calcium.

Food	Portion	Calcium (in mg)	% of RDA
Yogurt, plain, low-fat	1 cup	415	52
Sardines, Atlantic, drained solids	3 ounces	371	46
Mozzarella cheese, part-skim	2 ounces	366	46
Ricotta cheese, part-skim	½ cup	337	42
Mustard spinach, raw	1 cup, chopped	315	39
Milk, skim	1 cup	302	38
Milk, low-fat (1%)	1 cup	300	37
Salmon, Sockeye, drained solids	3 ounces	274	34
Collards, raw	1 cup, chopped	218	27
Chicory greens, raw	1 cup, chopped	180	22
Rhubarb, cooked	½ cup	174	22
Mustard spinach, cooked	½ cup, chopped	142	18
Amaranth, cooked	½ cup	138	17
Blackstrap molasses	1 tablespoon	137	17
Soybeans, green, cooked	½ cup	131	16
Tahini, roasted & toasted kernels	2 tablespoons	128	16
Cherimoyas	1 medium	126	16
Tahini, raw kernels	2 tablespoons	126	16
Spinach, cooked	½ cup	122	15
Tofu (soybean curd)	3 ounces	109	14
Turnip greens, cooked	½ cup, chopped	99	12
Kale, raw	1 cup, chopped	90	11
Broccoli, cooked	½ cup, chopped	89	11
Okra, cooked	½ cup, sliced	88	11
Figs, dried	3 medium	81	10
Oysters, raw	6 medium	81	10

The reason I have such wonderful success in reducing blood pressure in my patients is that the Mollen Method is tailor-made to promoting good health. It contains all the ingredients that scientific studies have shown are needed to stabilize blood pressure, such as:

• **Low salt**—The first thing any doctor tells a high blood pressure patient to do is cut down on salt. That's because studies have found that people with high blood pressure have more sodium in the walls of their blood vessels than do people with normal blood pressure.

• **High potassium**—Vegetables, fruits and fish are the mainstay of the diet. They are also rich sources of potassium, which helps blunt sodium's effect on blood pressure.

• **High calcium**—Studies have found that high blood pressure patients who increase their calcium intake decrease their blood pressure levels.

• **Weight loss**—As weight comes down, so, too, does blood pressure. Since the diet is low in fat, weight loss is a natural result.

• **Daily exercise**—Studies suggest that exercise has a definite positive effect on reducing blood pressure. The reason, according to one theory, is that exercise increases the body's ability to shift fluids out of circulation and into spaces between cells, causing the volume of blood to decrease and blood pressure to go down.

• **Moderate drinking**—Drinking alcohol raises blood pressure by weakening the kidneys and stiffening the arteries. A survey of 83,947 people in the United States found that those who drank three or more drinks a day had higher blood pressure than those who drank two or less drinks a day.

Angina Pain Eased

Angina pectoris, a condition characterized by chest and arm pains, is caused by insufficient oxygen in the heart muscles. Studies have shown that exercise, because of its amazing ability to facilitate oxygenation, can significantly reduce the number of angina attacks. The level of physical activity, of course, will be determined by a person's pain threshold. If angina pain occurs when your pulse rate hits 100, for instance, you should then exercise at a lower pulse rate.

As in other heart diseases, diet plays a crucial role in treatment. Body fats and cholesterol levels must be reduced.

Rex was 70 when he first came to see me with angina pain and high blood pressure. Rex, who had not even expected to live past 60, told me he was living on borrowed time. He also told me he couldn't follow the Mollen Method. A life of exercise and little red meat was just not his style. He was persistent but so was I. I finally got him to agree to give it a try. Where is he today, just one year later? Doing 10K races every other week. Instead of talking about how lucky he was to live past the magic number of 60, he talks about his plans for his 100th birthday!

Circulation Improved

Intermittent claudication is a circulatory condition caused by decreased circulation to the legs. Symptoms are severe pain and muscle cramps. Oddly enough, exercise can either improve or worsen the pain. I've found that a low-intensity daily walking program has helped my patients with this condition. The walking helps improve circulation in the legs. And the low-fat diet provides relief from muscle cramps and leg pain.

A more common circulatory problem is varicose veins. If you've been suffering from varicose veins or using them as an excuse not to exercise, it's time to change your thinking. Exercise may be the best thing for you. Of course, exercise won't make varicose veins disappear. However, it will help improve circulation in the lower extremities, preventing the pooling of blood and facilitating blood flow. The exercise and diet combined can help to prevent the progression of unsightly varicose veins.

Keep Blood Sugar under Control

In recent years many studies have suggested that a diet high in complex carbohydrates and low in fat can control blood sugar more effectively, thus reducing the possibility of developing diabetes and also helping to control hypoglycemia (low blood sugar). The complex carbohydrates contribute to a more controlled glucose absorption through the bowel, allowing insulin to be released more regularly. This high complex carbohydrate diet is the antithesis of the diet previously recommended for hypoglycemia, which in the past was based on high protein.

Since my diet minimizes fats and refined sugars, it plays a big role in controlling blood sugar. So it only makes sense that it is a good diet in helping to control diabetes.

But I've discovered that the exercise component may be even more important in controlling the disease than diet. That's because exercise improves the body's glucose utilization and decreases the amount of insulin that it demands. I have had several patients with blood sugar counts of more than 300 (70 to 120 is normal) who were able to control their blood sugar levels without medication. A strict program of diet and exercise stabilizes the body's sugar demand. In addition, it results in lower body weight, which is also important in improving a diabetic condition.

Some patients requiring injectable insulin have even been able to reduce the amount of insulin they need after going on the Mollen Method. In fact, one of my most remarkable patients is Rachel, who, at age 70, had a blood sugar count of 320 and was taking injectable insulin. I was able to control her diabetes with the Mollen Method. Her blood sugar is now normal and she no longer requires insulin or any other medication.

Fighting Depression

Depression. It's all part of being human. For some people, however, depression is more than an occasional state; it's a serious psychological problem. I don't think it's a coincidence at all that people who are affected with deep depression are often physically inactive people. When patients come to me complaining of depression I don't give them a prescription for pills to elevate their moods; I give them a prescription for exercise. If they would just move their bodies, I say, they will leave their depression behind. And I am by no means alone in this opinion.

In recent years, regular exercise has been one of the key treatments for depression. The theory is that the body gets a positive biochemical reaction from aerobic exercise. Exercise has been found to produce a benefit similar to antidepressant drugs.

Take Gloria. When Gloria first came to see me she was quite overweight and very depressed. After a month and a half, she had lost 35 pounds and her mental and emotional outlook had improved tenfold.

This is what Gloria had to say about the Mollen regimen: "I'm one of those dropouts; I'd tried everything. I thought, here I go, spending more money. I have spent thousands of dollars over 20 years trying to lose weight.

"I'd been to see three other doctors who put me on medications for high blood pressure, to lose weight and finally for depression. Dr. Mollen took me off all medication and had me start walking. At first I thought I was going to die.

"Today I'm a new person because of the Mollen Method. I'm a positive, not negative, person."

Why is regular exercise so deeply satisfying to the innermost person in each of us? No one knows for sure, but what is known is that exercise can alter your state of mind. One theory is that aerobic exercise releases endorphins—those chemicals in the brain that I told you are so important in reducing pain. Endorphins are also credited for eliciting what is known as the "runner's high"—that feeling runners say helps them "go the distance." Although this is still speculative, there are plenty of exercisers around (in fact, almost every exerciser I know!) who will attest to gaining psychological benefits from exercise. One such person is our friend Pat, who had this to say:

"I was always hiding behind my fat. I was just depressed all the time and didn't realize it. I didn't feel bad—I just didn't know what feeling good was like.

"I never had direct eye contact with anyone when I was heavier. Now I look people directly in the eye to make sure they have eye contact with me. My confidence, pride and self-respect have risen higher than I thought they ever could.

"If anyone ever gets depressed, they should just try the Mollen Method for 30 days to start feeling good again. I know it's difficult for depressed people to believe what I'm saying, but it really works. I wouldn't have believed it either. As they say, 'Try it. You'll like it.'"

Here is the Mollen antidepression prescription:

- Exercise for at least ten minutes daily.
- Participate in community projects.
- Talk to friends for at least 30 minutes a day.
- Eat a diet high in complex carbohydrates.
- Drink fruit juices (six ounces) at least six times daily.
- Avoid alcohol.
- Avoid fats.

The antidepression diet is effective. I recommend *no* alcohol because I find that depressed people often turn to alcohol. And since alcohol itself is a depressant, it only makes matters worse. So, if you've used alcohol as a crutch and want to get off, drink fruit juices six times daily in order to maintain a slightly elevated blood sugar level. This helps replace the sugar you got from alcohol (a lower blood sugar may contribute to depression). In addition, the complex carbohydrates will facilitate better control of blood sugar and decrease appetite. You should avoid high fats in the diet because they only cause sluggishness and fatigue which help to depress you.

Although the diet part of the Mollen Method will help to fight depression, in reality the exercise is the essential component. As I said, no one really knows why it works, they just know that it does. Who knows. Maybe it's just magic!

An Alcoholic's Story

David was a 38-year-old vice-president of a major corporation. He was also an alcoholic. He'd tried to quit several times with no success.

I didn't know David had a drinking problem when he first came to see me. He was 6'3" and 240 pounds and only said he was tired of having "the body of King Kong and the muscle tone of Twiggy." I told David I couldn't make him into Arnold Schwarzenegger, however I could help him lose weight and increase his muscle tone. He agreed and started the Mollen Method.

After 30 days, David was hooked. He was exercising every day and following the diet religiously. But it wan't until six weeks after our initial meeting that he confessed he was an alcoholic. He said he had not had a drink for two weeks and expressed amazement that his desire for alcohol had gradually been reduced through the exercise and diet.

David continued on the Mollen Method and by the end of six months he was down to 190 pounds (a 50-pound loss), which was perfect on his 6'3" frame. Since then, he has maintained his abstinence from alcohol and is finding that the Mollen Method helps him reduce the stress and strains of his job. He has not gained back any weight or had a drink.

David is by no means an isolated case. I have successfully treated many patients with alcoholism. Excessive drinking is often a negative response to stress, a nonproductive way of dealing with tension and anxiety. By gradually reducing the intake of alcohol and substituting exercise, my patients are given a new, *positive* stress release. Now, instead of being addicted to alcohol, these patients are addicted to exercise. I suggest the exercise be done first thing in the morning to help suppress any need for alcohol later in the day.

But there is something in the diet, too, that helps guard against the need for alcohol—fruit. Fruit compensates for the high sugar content that the alcohol once provided.

Obviously, the Mollen Method is not going to cure all the alcoholics in the world. However, it can be an excellent tool in the treatment of alcoholism when used in conjunction with a support group and professional counseling. Again, as in the treatment of depression, the exercise component is of paramount importance.

No More Ulcers

Jim had been an auto mechanic for 25 years. He was 49 and had not exercised since he was in high school. Periodically he had problems with an ulcer, which he tried to control by taking antacids. He believed his ulcer was something he'd just have to live with . . . until he awoke one night and began to spit up blood. He still had severe stomach pain when he came to see me the next day.

"Jim, if your car needed work, where would you take it?" I asked after I'd examined him.

"Well, I'm the best mechanic in town; I'd do the work myself," he answered.

"Well, you're also the best mechanic for your body," I said. I explained to Jim that he had to work on his body.

For the next three months, Jim exercised every day for at least ten minutes by walking, bicycling or jogging. He followed the diet, making sure he got plenty of fiber, very little fat and a minimal amount of protein. He gave up all rich and fried foods.

The regimen worked. It's been a year now and Jim has not had any problems with his ulcer, has lost weight and is no longer taking antacids. Again, the Mollen Method proved to be more valuable than medication in the treatment of disease.

Why had this diet worked when his regular eating routine hadn't? Because this diet is high in fiber, which causes the food to pass out of the stomach (where it can be an irritant) more quickly and into the bowel.

And Jim's not the only one to attest to the benefits of exercise for relieving symptoms. At the Honolulu Marathon Clinic, athletes reported a lessening of gastrointestinal problems, ulcers and hemorrhoids as a result of their vigorous exercise schedule.

Here is my anti-ulcer regimen:

- Exercise daily for ten minutes.
- Eat plenty of fiber foods.
- Steam all vegetables.
- Avoid all spices.
- Avoid high doses of vitamin C.
- Avoid antacids.
- Avoid caffeine.
- Avoid all rich foods, including shellfish (lobster, crab, shrimp) and chocolate.

Menopause–the Easy Way

Of all the diseases and discomforts that I have treated with exercise and diet, few demonstrate more positive results than those experienced by women going through menopause. Complaints of discomfort are minimized as adherence to the Mollen Method is maximized. Why?

Because exercise improves circulation, which is often slowed down during "the change." A reduction in sugar and caffeine consumption helps reduce the number of hot flashes, making it possible for many women to reduce, if not eliminate, their dependence on Estrogen Replacement Therapy (ERT). ERT, which carries its own set of side effects, is often used to treat hot flashes. In addition, patients have reported a better mental attitude. The loss of weight and inches helps contribute to this state of well-being, making some patients exclaim that they've never felt better in years. (Honest!)

But the real benefit of diet and exercise is the role they play in warding off osteoporosis, the disease of "brittle bones" that strikes one out of every four women beyond the age of 45.

Exercise is imperative in the battle against osteoporosis. Studies show that exercise enhances bone strength. Also important to healthy bones is calcium. As a woman ages, her need for calcium increases. Although the Recommended Dietary Allowance is 800 milligrams, women in their menopausal years and postmenopausal years should make sure they get more–at least 1,500 milligrams a day. (For a list of foods high in calcium, turn to page 32.) In fact, I feel calcium is so important, I recommend that women take calcium supplements daily to insure they get their daily dose.

Exercise Improves Asthma

Asthmatics think they have a built-in excuse not to exercise: "My doctor says I can't." Well, I'm one doctor (and I know there are others) who says you can.

Asthmatics actually respond quite well to exercise, but they must exercise at a lower intensity than nonasthmatics. So don't be so quick to jump into that rocker and rock yourself into disease. I won't let you off the hook that easily. You'll have to give me more excuses, and prize-winning ones at that, to avoid the Mollen Method. Simply saying "I have asthma" won't do it.

In fact, in 1980 I put on a race for asthmatic children. Everyone thought that I was crazy recommending exercise for asthmatic children. The response, however, was overwhelmingly positive—both from the children and their parents. Today, there are many pulmonary experts throughout the country who recommend exercise routinely for the treatment of asthma.

Exercise not only helps to improve the tone of the breathing muscles, but strengthens the cardiovascular system as well. Exercise also encourages patients to stop smoking by providing an alternate mechanism for dealing with stress.

Children who are asthmatic do even better on an exercise program than adults. This is because their lungs are not as affected by the disease process, nor are they as contaminated by tobacco as the lungs of adults.

Most asthmatic children do well in an indoor swimming program because of the pollen-free environment. Bobby, age 13, was one of these. I told him to swim 10 lengths a day. Within a period of two months, he was swimming 100 lengths, as well as doing 20 push-ups and 30 sit-ups on a daily basis. This exercise not only improved his overall mental attitude and self-confidence, it enhanced his posture and muscle tone as well.

In addition to the exercise program, Bobby was placed on a diet that eliminated dairy products, corn and wheat—allergens that often affect asthmatics. His symptoms were thereby reduced, making possible a decrease in medication. Whether all of an asthmatic's medication can be eliminated with the Mollen Method depends upon the severity of the disease.

If exercise-induced asthma is your problem, I'd suggest using an inhaler (albuterol) prior to exercise to reduce the severity of attacks. It's most important to exercise at a low intensity, trying to avoid elevating your pulse rate above 120 beats per minute, or 70 percent of your maximum level.

An Alternative to Surgery

You have two choices as to how you can spend this weekend—go for a long walk or be admitted to the hospital for surgery. Which do you prefer? Silly question, I know. But if more people would spend more time walking (or doing any kind of exercise) they could reduce their chances of ever having surgery.

For example, Ken, 26, was jogging one day when his knee suddenly gave out. He had never been bothered by knee pain, had never played football or been in an accident. Yet, Ken was told that his right knee had a torn cartilage (the stabilizing tissue of the internal part of the knee) and that surgery should be done immediately.

Ken declined surgery for the time being and decided to see me.

Instead of surgery, I started Ken on stretching and strengthening exercises for his knee. I had him walk several miles daily. In two months Ken was again jogging two miles a day. There was no pain, no swelling and no discomfort in his knee. And, he never had surgery.

Then there is Judy. At 45 she was suffering from an aching lower back. The pain was controlled by taking several Percodan and four doses of Valium a day. After three months on the medication, she was getting only minimal relief. Then she was told she had a ruptured disc and needed a laminectomy, the surgical removal of a disc between the fourth and fifth lumbar vertebrae.

Judy refused surgery and came to see me. I couldn't reverse a ruptured disc, but I knew I could minimize the disc problem with a prescription of exercise, diet and weight loss.

Initially, I prescribed stretching exercises and abdominal exercises to compensate for the weak back muscles. The stretching exercises improved the flexibility of the muscles in Judy's lower back, relieving some of the pressure from the ruptured disc. She started walking every day and ultimately lost 30 pounds. She now experiences occasional pain only from prolonged standing on hard-surfaced floors, and she is addicted to exercise as she was once addicted to drugs.

Then there is Cindy, who at age 38 and 350 pounds had finally had it with being overweight. She was depressed by her inability to lose weight despite trying a variety of diets for ten years. The last doctor she visited had suggested that she have a partial gastric resection (stomach removal), which, she was informed, was only used in the most serious cases. Cindy agreed to have the surgery. However, 24 hours beforehand, she became apprehensive and came to see me. "Thank God I found you," she said.

Cindy has followed the Mollen Method for six months and has lost 60 pounds. She walks daily, follows the diet and has a more positive (and motivated) outlook on life. She is convinced that her lifestyle change—taking control of her life—is the only thing that could possibly have saved her.

And last but not least is George, a 51-year-old accountant who declined to have coronary bypass surgery for the blockage in his major coronary artery because, as he put it, "The economics of it just don't make sense."

The average coronary bypass costs at least $20,000. George, being the wise accountant he is, decided to come see me instead. At the time, he was unable to walk a half block without severe chest pain. He was on heart medication. His initial weight was 225 pounds and his cholesterol count was a high 330. He had always concerned himself with the material things of life and the years had flown past him like the numbers on his calculator.

Now he was more concerned with his own physical being.

As incredible as it may sound, 30 days from the time that George came to my office, he had lost 25 pounds, was experiencing no chest pain, was taken off all medication and was walking two miles a day as well as riding a stationary bicycle the equivalent of ten miles a day. Now, his cholesterol count has dropped to 170 and he has had a total change in attitude toward life. The Mollen Method of diet and exercise was just the right prescription for him!

George is proud of the fact that he saved $20,000 by not having surgery. He considers this the best investment of his life.

The stories can go on and on. Maybe you have one of your own. Diet and exercise are powerful prescriptions for many ailments. When you get the feeling something is getting you down, it's no time to give up on your program. Just remember, exercise today can keep you from more serious problems tomorrow.

Slow the Aging Process

I can honestly say that at this point in medical history, there is no greater contributor to renewed health than daily exercise combined with a natural, low-fat diet. It also may be the prescription for a longer life. The aging process, along with its attendant catalogue of woes, can be significantly slowed with proper diet and exercise. For example, look at the Tarahumara Indians of northern Mexico whose longevity ranges from 100 to 120 years of age. They exercise regularly and hold ceremonial runs of 100 miles. Their diet consists mostly of corn and beans. Heart disease and high blood pressure are foreign to their society. We can't ignore this fact. Our consciences and survival instincts can't allow us to believe it's mere coincidence.

There is also a group of people in northern Russia who walk up and down a hill five miles each way to work each day. They, too, have a low incidence of heart disease and high blood pressure. The common denominator in these societies is daily exercise.

On the other hand, the Japanese people have had a low incidence of heart disease for years which has been related to their low-fat diet. However, Japanese people living in the United States who have become accustomed to a Western diet have the same share of heart disease as Americans.

I won't belabor the point. Exercise and diet will make a difference in your life and reduce the risk of developing the common degenerative diseases of our society in later years.

Independence from Disease

To paraphrase Thomas Jefferson, one of the founding fathers of our country, you should devote at least two hours a day to bodily exercise and, if you do not want to, later on in life you will devote at least two hours a day to disease. Jefferson was not only responsible for the Declaration of Independence but was also one of the first to declare what it takes to be independent from disease. So I suggest you take a tip from our erudite forefather.

Start with the minimal addictive dose of ten minutes a day of exercise for the next 30 days. Begin a low-fat diet. With this program you'll be on your way to a disease-free life.

Some people are simply more susceptible to disease than others. Medical science is unsure why this is true. But what we do know is that the higher our resistance the less susceptible we are to disease. In addition, evidence suggests regular exercise and a proper diet, including minimal alcohol consumption and no smoking, can increase our resistance and lessen our susceptibility to disease.

So the choice is yours. You can devote time to exercise daily, follow proper diet guidelines and make lifestyle changes now or be compelled later on in life to devote several hours a day to nursing your disease.

Chapter 4

EXERCISE – TEN MINUTES A DAY

The proverbial monkey on the back of Americans these days is the tire around their middles: flab. I can't think of a battle that is more pervasive or persistently frustrating than the fight to deflate that tire. The Fight against Flab is a two-weapon war. Yet, most overweight Americans only use one.

The weapon they use is diet.

But why fight the war with a single weapon? Would you try to win a boxing match by using only one hand? You're limiting yourself to one kind of ammunition and that ammunition is sheer willpower.

In the Fight against Flab, willpower won't gain you any ground. Oh, you may succeed in shedding some pounds, but how long will they stay off? Anyone who's tried it knows that it's not for long.

It's a no-win situation. You go on a crash diet. You lose the weight. You're happy. Then you go back to your old eating routine, and before long you regain the old weight. You're unhappy. Then you begin yet another diet. It's a battle that is neverending, never won.

But you won't go through this on the Mollen Method. And that's what separates my diet from other weight-loss programs. My entire concept of health is twofold. It takes diet *and* exercise to make it work.

If you put energy into the body in the form of food, you must work it back out in the form of exercise. It's that simple. If you don't work to get rid of the food you eat, the body will store it in the form of fat. And the excess fat will form another roll around your middle or an extra chin hanging from your face.

So when people ask, "Should I exercise every day?" I always answer by asking, "Do you plan to eat every day?" If you put energy in, you've got to take it out, no matter how much–or how little–you eat.

Why Dieting Alone Doesn't Work

In fact, depending on diet alone to lose weight actually works against you. You become hungry, grumpy and out-of-sorts. Your energy level takes a dive simply because you're trying to survive on portions that wouldn't keep a parakeet happy. Dieting becomes a negative experience because you're depriving yourself of one of the things you love most–food. (After all, if you didn't love food you wouldn't have a weight problem, would you?)

Your whole body rebels when you deprive it of food. As you cut your intake of food down, down, you also slow your metabolism down, down. Your body begins to think you're caught in a famine and, in an effort to keep you from starving to death, lowers the rate at which it burns food. So if you have a slow metabolism to begin with, dieting makes it even slower.

Exercise, on the other hand, has the opposite effect on metabolism. Exercise can actually stoke a low-burning metabolism. Not only is your metabolism working extra duty while you exercise, it keeps on burning for hours after you've stopped, even while you're sleeping!

And don't try to come back at me with the excuse that exercise will only make you eat more. Sorry, but that excuse just doesn't hold water. I rarely have patients who complain of being hungry on my program. In fact, there is even scientific research to back up the claim that exercise doesn't increase hunger. A group of overweight women was brought into a clinic, ostensibly so that researchers could moderate their metabolic rate. They didn't know the real reason for the experiment–to measure how much they would eat after exercising. For 19 days they were left to sit and do nothing; they were allowed to eat at will. Then, for the next 19 days they were put on a daily exercise program. Again they were allowed to eat whenever they wanted to. But they ate no more when they exercised than when they didn't. Exercise didn't make them any hungrier!

BENEFITS OF EXERCISE

Restrict your food intake and you end up with one nice benefit from your weeks of effort—weight loss. But add exercise to your reducing pro-gram and you'll find the benefits mushrooming. Some of the most obvious will be:

- More weight loss
- Less fat and bulge, more muscle
- Greater lung capacity
- Reduced risk of heart disease
- Improved mental attitude
- More energy
- Improved sleeping patterns
- Improved complexion
- Improved bowel function
- Reduced irritability and anxiety
- Stress control
- Improved creativity
- Improved productivity
- Increased self-confidence

The Body Fat Factor

There's one more thing that exercise can do for you that dieting alone can't. And this is perhaps the most important thing of all.

Exercise burns fat and builds muscle. Dieting doesn't. In fact, the opposite is true. When people diet without the benefit of exercise, they burn muscle along with fat. Some 30 percent of their initial weight loss comes from muscle. That's why many of the people you see who've gone on quick-weight-loss diets look so gaunt and saggy. They're losing too much of the good and not enough of the bad. They may end up a little thinner, but they'll also end up a little flabbier.

But add exercise to your food-control program, and you'll find a brand-new you. You'll be leaner and firmer. Your belly that once felt like a water balloon will become tight and flat. Your complexion will take on a healthy look. You'll look better than you ever did in your life. Your friends will tell you, your clothes will tell you, your mirror will tell you! Eventually you'll even find that counting calories isn't as important as it was in the past. That's because muscle has still another advantage over fat—it burns calories faster than fat does.

All this explains a lot about the way we look as we age—if we don't exercise. Sure, you may be one of the "lucky" few who doesn't lift a finger to exercise yet hasn't gained a pound since you graduated from high school or college 15 years ago. But I dare you to try on the blue jeans you used to wear in those days. You'll most likely find they don't fit the way they used to. In fact, you may find that they don't fit at all.

Can this be true, you say? Can I really stay the same weight but get broader at the same time? Yes! It simply means you've been trading in lean body muscle for fat. Some people like to call it middle-age spread. I call it inactivity. That explains why two women can be the same height and each weigh 120 pounds, yet one is a size 8 and the other is a 12. One has more muscle and the other has more fat. Muscle weighs more than fat but takes up less room.

So, even if you aren't overweight, you can be overfat and out of shape. That means it's time you got on the Mollen Method, too.

How much body fat should you have? The average American male is about 15 to 18 percent body fat, and the average American female is about 22 to 24 percent body fat. This is way too high. I suggest that my male patients get down to 10 to 15 percent fat and females to 15 to 18 percent fat.

A Healthy Heart

Ask most people what finally motivated them to go out and exercise and they most likely will tell you "to lose a little weight." If they mention for "the health of it" at all, it usually comes in second. That's fine. For even if your sole reason for exercising is weight loss, you can't help but benefit from what I consider equally important—cardiovascular conditioning. While no one can guarantee you won't develop a heart condition or suffer a heart attack sometime in your life, the Mollen Method will help you reduce the odds.

As I mentioned in Chapter 1, aerobic activity will make your heart stronger. That is because your heart is a muscle. Like any muscle in the body, if you put it to work you can increase its size. Increase the size of a muscle and you'll increase its output. Your heart will be able to pump out more blood with each beat. When you're at rest, your heart will be at rest, too, pumping much slower, saving itself wear and tear. When you climb a flight of stairs, for example, your heart will manage the stress more efficiently. It won't require as many beats to pump out the same amount of blood and oxygen to the rest of your body as it would if you were not in good condition. It makes that trip up so much easier. You won't gasp for a breath at the top of the first flight; you'll just head for the second without giving it extra thought. An unconditioned heart must work twice as hard as the conditioned heart.

For example, my resting pulse is 50 beats per minute. If your pulse is 80 beats per minute at rest, when you go up a flight of stairs or climb a hill, your heart rate might elevate to 160 beats per minute. But my heart rate will elevate to only 100 beats per minute. I'll save my heart undue wear and tear because I'm in better shape than you are. You can't help but build a healthy heart—and a healthy life—when you take up exercise.

That Feel-Good Feeling

Ah, exercise can do such wonderful things for you! It can slim you down, giving you that urge to look in the mirror (instead of avoiding it) and loving what you see—the waist you lost ten years ago, thinner thighs, a flatter stomach. It can give you a stronger heart, one that can take you long

---

AIM HIGH TO REACH LOW

To be aerobic, an exercise must place a reasonable amount of stress on your heart and lungs. It must push your heart rate high and keep it there for a sustained period of time.

The payoff? A lower heart rate when you aren't exercising. When you're not exercising (which is most of the day), your heart will beat more slowly, saving it wear and tear over a lifetime. When you're under stress or an emergency hits and your heart begins to pound (sometimes at twice its normal rate), it will race more slowly, too, keeping it out of the danger zone and preventing undue stress or possibly even a heart attack.

For the best aerobic workout you should raise your resting pulse rate to at least 70 percent, but not more than 85 percent, of its maximum. It's always important to monitor your heart rate because you don't want to get it too high (this could be dangerous) or allow it to remain too low (which means you aren't getting much of a workout at all).

You can measure your heart rate simply by counting your pulse for 60 seconds, either in your neck (carotid), your head (temporal) or your wrist (radial).

Your exercise pulse rate is considered 70 percent of maximum. To measure this, take 220 minus your age and multiply by 70 percent. Your maximum pulse rate is 85 percent. To measure this, take 220 minus your age and multiply by 85 percent. For example, if you're age 30, you'd figure out your heart rate as follows:

$$220 - 30 = 190 \times .70 = 133$$
$$220 - 30 = 190 \times .85 = 162$$

distances without wearing you down. But there's more—something you never really bargained for. You'll feel better than you ever have in your entire life. Exercise will put into your life that bounce that you haven't experienced since you were a school kid. It'll have you looking for activity instead of an easy chair when you're at a family outing.

Exercise will leave you feeling good about yourself and the things around you. Your self-confidence will grow as your body whittles down. The stresses of every day will gradually become less stressful. You'll feel healthy and in control of your life. That's what the Mollen Method is all about—a new lifestyle.

You remember my patient Pat who has maintained a weight loss of 90 pounds for the first time in her life? Why did the Mollen Method work for her when every other diet she tried in the past failed? Simply the addition of exercise. "Without a doubt, the exercise is what made the difference for me," says Pat.

"I always used to avoid exercise like the plague. I used all the excuses—I'm exhausted from working, or I don't have the time. But now if I don't exercise, I feel guilty. Exercise makes me feel so much better and gives me more energy. I can't stand it when I don't exercise.

"It's the most important part of my weight control and I realize it has to be an integral part of my life forever."

Exercise is a catch-22: If you don't exercise you feel tired and you don't want to exercise at all. On the other hand, if you do exercise your energy level soars.

Then there's Julia Firestone. Exercise also made a dramatic change in her life. My first encounter with Julia occurred when she was walking rather timidly with her housekeeper down the road close to my home. I gave her a grand "hello" but only got a meek response. I later learned that "Lady Julia," as she is affectionately referred to by her closest friends, had recently lost her husband, Peter, of the well-known Firestone tire family.

Lady Julia and I were eventually introduced and became good friends. I subtly encouraged her to start jogging regularly. It wasn't long before Julia was jogging three to four miles daily with longer runs on the weekend. But it wasn't the jogger she became that was the most remarkable change in Julia. It was the way she felt about herself. In Lady Julia's words, "I feel more self-confident. I like myself better and my body feels more toned and tight. It's like being given a gift of youth—you feel and look ten years younger almost instantly. The addiction to the Mollen Method was subtle, but precise! I feel sexier. It's a total feeling of being healthy. In fact, when your 18-year-old son starts telling you that you look younger and prettier, you definitely know that something must be working right."

I, too, can attest to the great feeling you can derive from exercise. In fact, it's what's made me an exercise addict.

I exercise every day. I run for an hour, bicycle for a half-hour and lift weights for another half-hour. On weekends I exercise even more. And I love it.

But it wasn't always that way. When I began running 15 years ago, I hated it. But there was something about it I liked immediately—the way it made me *feel*. I felt great after a run and I could actually feel my energy level increasing. I ran two miles a day for months. Then, I realized that I could change that by running more slowly and perhaps longer. I advanced to four miles a day. I could breathe, talk and run at the same time. I lost 25 pounds over the next three months. My mental attitude improved, the stress came under control, I became more self-confident. My cholesterol level (originally 270) came down to 130. At this point I realized that a lifestyle of health and fitness can be fun. I was hooked. And I want the same thing to happen to you.

Easing into Exercise

For the next 30 days I want exercise to become your new source of nourishment. You'd probably never think of skipping a meal, would you? For the next 30 days I don't want you to skip a day of exercise. I ask that because I want to make *you* an exercise addict, too. All it takes is ten minutes a day. It's the minimal addictive dose.

You say it can't happen to you? You're wrong. I know, right now walking sounds like a lot of work. But do as I ask for 30 days and you'll be hooked. Try to give it up after that and I guarantee you'll experience depression, anxiety, irritability, insomnia and fatigue. In short, all the same symptoms (but obviously less severe and traumatic) you'd have if you were addicted to a drug like heroin and attempted to give it up cold turkey. Stick with the exercise, however, and you'll not only experience a natural high, but you'll keep going back for another dose, day after day.

You will build endurance as you go along. You'll start easy and build slowly. As time goes by you'll naturally add minutes to your endurance. Your body will adjust. The result will be that before you know it, you'll be doing things you never imagined possible—as well as losing weight and inches, and feeling good!

Stop shaking in your boots, and wipe the sweat from your brow. You will not be asked to run the Boston Marathon, swim the English Channel or bike the Tour de France. I am not interested in making you a "world-class athlete," simply a "world-class health enthusiast."

Just ten minutes a day of exercise every day for the next 30 days. After that time if you don't feel better, look better and haven't lost any weight, you can go back to the other dozen or so quick-weight-loss remedies that have failed you in the past. But I need a commitment from you for a *full* 30 days. It's the only way to make the Mollen Method work.

First, let's clarify what I mean by exercise. I want you to do some type of aerobic exercise—the kind that gets your heart pumping and the sweat flowing—for at least ten minutes every day. By this I mean exercise like running, bicycling, swimming, aerobic dancing, jumping rope and, yes, even walking. There's an entire list of aerobic exercise schedules you can follow on pages 62-104. Choose one. Choose several. Just make sure you do *something* and do it *every day*.

Sure, you say. This might be easy enough for some people. But what about those who have done nothing more strenuous in the past ten years than bring in the groceries? Where do they begin?

I don't mean to sound like a smart alec, but I'll tell you. You begin by placing one foot in front of the other and *start moving.*

Now I know that you know deep down inside that exercise is something you really need. Most likely it's also something you'd probably really like to do, but you just don't know the right way to go about it.

Oh, you've tried, you say. And failed. Well, that only means you've taken on too much, too fast. That's the downfall of most exercise dropouts. That's why I'm starting you out *slowly*.

If you've never exercised before, of if you're very overweight and find other activities too difficult, walking is the ideal starting point. But let's get something straight right from the start—I don't mean *strolling*. I've already told you that the ten minutes of exercise I'm requiring from you each day is heavy duty—aerobic. The kind that keeps you huffing and puffing and raises your heart rate. The kind that puts swing in your arms when you're walking.

If you're a little sheepish about the whole thing I suggest you go to a local shopping center or mall, where you'll be among many walkers. Measure the distance from one end of the mall to the other and then walk the distance you're supposed to cover that day. (This will also keep you from using weather as an excuse not to exercise.)

Of course, walking isn't your only choice. If you're already good at keeping on the move at a good clip, you might try to spend your ten-minute workout doing my favorite kind of exercise, running. By mixing walking and jogging you can easily turn yourself into a full-time runner by the end of your 30 days. Who knows. Some day I may meet you in a marathon!

FOOD EQUIVALENCIES OF CERTAIN EXERCISES

1 mile jogging = 100 calories = 1 apple

3 to 4 miles bicycling = 100 calories = 1 tablespoon butter

10 minutes swimming = 100 calories = 1 slice toast with butter

40 to 60 minutes singles tennis = 100 calories = ½ cup cottage cheese

90 to 120 minutes golf = 150 calories = 1 12-ounce bottle of beer

20 to 30 minutes racquetball = 100 calories = ½ cup ice cream

Choosing an Exercise

I realize I'm a bit prejudiced, but I consider jogging to be the best exercise there is. Not because I've run 30 marathons, participated in 5 triathlons and written the book *Run for Your Life* (Doubleday, 1978), but because jogging simply provides the most benefits in the shortest period of time. For instance, most people can run one mile in 10 minutes. One mile of jogging burns 100 calories. That's equal to 15 minutes on the minitrampoline, 13 minutes on the stationary bicycle, 20 minutes of walking, 30 minutes of aerobic dancing and 4 hours of pond fishing or card playing. So in terms of getting the most exercise for your money, 10 minutes a day, jogging is about the best you can do.

And forget what others tell you. Jogging isn't hard. Run at a comfortable pace, one in which you can hold a conversation and one that doesn't leave you panting. Believe it or not, if it's done slowly without elevating your pulse too high and causing breathlessness, it can be easy. You see, heavy breathing should be saved for the likes of Carl Lewis, the Olympic sprinter who runs 100 meters as fast and as hard as he can and does it in record time. Labored breathing has no place in your exercise arena, at least not in the beginning. Of course, I won't be upset if you don't take up jogging (a little disappointed, but not upset). I realize there are other aerobic activities you might enjoy more, like bicycling, swimming or jumping rope.

I consider bicycling an excellent choice. Three miles of bicycling outdoors equals a mile of jogging. (Forgive me, but I have a habit of comparing everything to jogging.) Of course, it depends on the intensity of your ride. For the person who wants to use a stationary bicycle, four or five miles equals a mile of jogging. That's with the tension set for about 20 miles an hour and maintaining a pulse at 120 beats per minute.

If you favor swimming, keep in mind that 10 minutes of swimming equals about a mile of jogging (that's figuring you can swim a mile in 30 minutes). A mile of swimming equals about three miles of jogging.

A word about swimming. It is good exercise, but don't expect to burn as many calories swimming as you would riding a bicycle or jogging. Because you're in the water, swimming doesn't allow your body temperature (and therefore, your metabolism) to increase like it does during sweat-producing exercise. Of course, how efficiently you do burn calories while swimming will depend upon your own metabolism and your physical condition. For some people, swimming is an excellent exercise.

Other excellent exercises from which you can choose are walking, jumping rope, stair climbing, the minitrampoline, the rowing machine, aerobic dance, hiking and cross-country skiing.

Although other exercises such as tennis, racquetball and squash may elevate your pulse rate, they seldom sustain the elevation for a continued period of time. However, if played vigorously and regularly they may be beneficial, providing the cardiovascular and calorie-burning effects that are necessary. If you play such a sport one or two days a week you can substitute an hour of play for your ten minutes of exercise that day, should you care to.

Which exercise you choose makes little difference to me as long as it's aerobic. The aerobic effect of exercise will not only provide physical benefits but mental, emotional and spiritual benefits as well.

Why Sporadic Exercise Doesn't Work

Some people will say, "Wait, I played baseball today, doesn't that count? Afer all, I was out there for *three* hours." Sure, you were out there three hours, but how much time did you spend actually doing *strenuous* activity? Maybe 20 minutes of those three hours? And even those 20 minutes—when you were running the bases or chasing the ball—were not a

(Continued on page 59)

THE MOLLEN MEASURE OF FITNESS

The number of calories burned during a particular activity doesn't necessarily reflect the benefits to your heart and circulation. Some activities require a lot of stops and starts or short bursts of energy; therefore, the heart rate is sometimes not sustained at an elevated level long enough to improve your aerobic capacity. In the chart below I've given an aerobic rating to some of the more popular activities.

The chart is based on the amount of calories burned by a 150-pound person. Calorie usage will vary slightly depending upon the weight of the individual. For every 10-pound difference you weigh above 150, add 7 calories to every 100. For every 10-pound difference below 150, subtract 7 calories. For example, if you weigh 130 pounds, basing your calculation on the chart below, you can figure that one mile of jogging is equivalent to consuming 86 calories. If you weigh 170 pounds, a mile of jogging burns about 114 calories.

1 - Excellent   3 - Fair
2 - Good   4 - Poor

Aerobic Rating	Exercise	Duration	Calories	Time Period	Comments
2	Aerobic dancing		100 200 300	= 30 min. = 60 min. = 90 min.	Depends upon the intensity of the class.
4	Archery		50 100 150	= 30 min. = 60 min. = 90 min.	Depends on number of arrows shot.
1	Backpacking	2 miles 4 miles	250 500	= 1 hour = 2 hours	Calories burned will vary depending on the uphill and downhill terrain. This is based on carrying a 25-pound pack.
3	Badminton	1 game 2 games 3 games	25 50 150	= 10 min. = 20 min. = 60 min.	This is based on singles play by players of equal ability.

Aerobic Rating	Exercise	Duration	Cal- ories	Time Period	Comments
3	Baseball	1 game	100	= 1 hour	Depends on amount of
		1 game	200	= 2 hours	base running.
		1 game	300	= 3 hours	
2	Basketball	1 game	100	= 20 min.	Count only the time in
		2 games	200	= 40 min.	which you are actively
		3 games	300	= 60 min.	involved.
1	Bicycling, outdoor	3 miles	100	= 10 min.	Hills can increase
		6 miles	200	= 20 min.	caloric output and car-
		12 miles	400	= 40 min.	diovascular endurance.
1	Bicycling, stationary	4 miles	100	= 13 min.	Varies with tension
		8 miles	200	= 26 min.	level and speed.
		16 miles	300	= 52 min.	
4	Bowling	3 games	60	= 1 hour	Weight of the ball
		6 games	120	= 2 hours	won't affect caloric
		9 games	180	= 3 hours	expenditure.
2	Boxing	5 rounds	250	= 15 min.	Varies with the aggres-
		10 rounds	500	= 30 min.	sion of the boxer.
		15 rounds	750	= 45 min.	
2	Calisthenics (push-ups, sit-ups, etc.)		50	= 10 min.	Count only the time
			100	= 20 min.	during which you
			150	= 30 min.	participate.
4	Driving car		50	= 1 hour	Will vary upon the
	Driving				amount of turns, stop-
	motorcycle		120	= 1 hour	ping and steering.
	Driving truck		80	= 1 hour	
3	Fencing	1 match	25	= 7.5 min.	
		2 matches	50	= 15 min.	
		3 matches	100	= 30 min.	
3	Golf	9 holes	75	= 1 hour	No motor carts
		18 holes	150	= 2 hours	allowed.
3	Gymnastics		100	= 20 min.	Count only time
			200	= 40 min.	exercising.
			300	= 60 min.	

(Continued)

THE MOLLEN MEASURE OF FITNESS – Continued

Aerobic Rating	Exercise	Duration	Cal- ories	Time Period	Comments
2	Handball	1 game 2 games 3 games	100 200 300	= 20 min. = 40 min. = 60 min.	Count only the time in which you are actively involved.
2	Hockey		100 200 300	= 20 min. = 40 min. = 60 min.	Count only the time in which you are actively participating.
4	Horseback riding		50 100	= 30 min. = 60 min.	Recreational riding is an excellent exercise– for the horse.
1	Jogging	1 mile 2 miles 3 miles	100 200 300	= 10 min. = 20 min. = 30 min.	Speed is relatively unimportant in num- ber of calories burned. Body weight is more important.
1	Jumping rope		75 150	= 5 to 8 min. = 10 to 15 min.	Skip with both feet together or step over the rope alternating one foot at a time.
2	Karate		100 200 300	= 20 min. = 40 min. = 60 min.	Will depend upon practice or match involvement.
1	Lacrosse & soccer	1 game 1 game 1 game	150 300 450	= 20 min. = 40 min. = 60 min.	Count only the time in which you are actively participating.
4	Motorcross		300 to 400	= 1 hour	Will vary with the amount of turns, stop- ping and steering.
3	Ping pong	3 games 6 games 9 games	75 150 225	= 30 min. = 60 min. = 90 min.	

Aerobic Rating	Exercise	Duration	Cal- ories	Time Period	Comments
2	Racquetball	1 game	100	= 20 min.	Count only the time in
		2 games	200	= 40 min.	which you are actively
		3 games	300	= 60 min.	involved.
1	Rebounder (mini- trampoline)		35	= 5 min.	Land heel to toe as if
			70	= 10 min.	jogging for maximal
			100	= 15 min.	benefits.
			135	= 20 min.	
1	Rowing machine		100	= 6 min.	Will depend upon the
			200	= 12 min.	intensity and number
			300	= 24 min.	of strokes per minute.
1	Running in place	700 steps	100	= 10 min.	Depends upon number
		1,400 steps	200	= 20 min.	of steps for every
		2,100 steps	300	= 30 min.	minute.
3	Skateboarding		30	= 15 min.	Will vary with the
			60	= 30 min.	terrain and the number
			120	= 60 min.	of hills involved.
1	Skating		100	= 30 min.	Either ice or roller
			200	= 60 min.	skating. For speed skating, the calories increase significantly.
2	Skiing (downhill)		100 to 150	= 30 min.	Count only actual skiing time. These
			200 to 300	= 60 min.	figures also apply to water skiing.
1	Skiing (cross- country)		200 to 300	= 30 min.	Cross-country skiing is considered the best
			400 to 600	= 60 min.	aerobic conditioner.
2	Squash	1 game	100	= 20 min.	Count only the time in
		2 games	200	= 40 min.	which you are actively
		3 games	300	= 60 min.	involved.

(Continued)

THE MOLLEN MEASURE OF FITNESS – *Continued*

Aerobic Rating	Exercise	Duration	Cal-ories	Time Period	Comments
1	Stair climbing		200	= 10 min.	Count only the time walking upstairs.
			600	= 30 min.	
			1,200	= 60 min.	
1	Swimming	400 meters	100	= 10 min.	Freestyle. However breaststroke and butterfly burn more calories.
		800 meters	200	= 20 min.	
		1,200 meters	300	= 30 min.	
3	Tennis	1 set	50	= 20 min.	Doubles uses up half the calories. Of course, calories burned depend upon intensity of play.
		2 sets	100	= 40 min.	
		3 sets	150	= 60 min.	
2	Touch football		200	= 30 min.	Count only the time in which you are actively participating.
			400	= 60 min.	
			600	= 90 min.	
3	Volleyball	1 game	100	= 30 min.	Count only the time in which you are actively participating.
		2 games	200	= 60 min.	
2	Walking	1 mile	100	= 20 min.	Speed is relatively unimportant in cal-ories burned; distance counts.
		2 miles	200	= 40 min.	
		3 miles	300	= 60 min.	
3	Weight lifting		100	= 30 min.	Count only the time lifting.
			200	= 60 min.	
			300	= 90 min.	
2	Wrestling		60	= 5 min.	Count only the time in which you are actively involved.
			120	= 10 min.	
			180	= 15 min.	
3	Yoga		25	= 10 min.	This is for Hatha Yoga. The meditational type will use fewer calories.
			50	= 20 min.	
			75	= 30 min.	

sustained effort. It was sporadic. So baseball may be fun, but it won't do you a bit of good if you're counting on it for aerobic exercise. As for weight loss—well, at least it keeps you out of the kitchen.

Even if you do aerobic exercise, but only do it once in a while (like once or twice a week), it isn't going to do you much good, either. Not only will it prevent you from becoming addicted to the Mollen Method, you will not burn a sufficient number of calories to lose weight.

Most people think that they're receiving more benefits from exercise than they are. For instance, the person who bowls three games believes they've burned at least 500 calories and are therefore entitled to a few beers as compensation for those efforts. And they often reward themselves with exactly that. Unfortunately, they burned less than 100 calories and received no cardiovascular conditioning—regardless of the weight of the ball they were carrying around.

You say you play golf? Golf is a great game and a great recreational sport, but it does little for your cardiovascular system. If you walked the perimeter of a golf course, you'd burn 300 calories, the equivalent of running three miles. But it is only 3/16th of a mile from hole to hole so you don't get sustained elevation of your pulse rate. And it might take you all morning to play that game of golf, but you could jog that three miles in 30 minutes!

Horseback riding is a great exercise—for the horse. It does very little for the person on top—unless you have a runaway horse. That would certainly give you a sustained pulse!

Finally, skydiving may be an excellent sport to elevate your pulse rate, but as a daily exercise for providing conditioning benefits, it ranks extremely low. In addition, the risk of injury and even death are significantly higher than in most aerobic exercises.

In fact, I have a friend, Tom, who is a professional skydiving instructor. I've been trying to convince Tom to run a marathon (26.2 miles), and he's been trying to get me to jump from a plane at 10,000 feet. He has suggested that he would run one-half a marathon (13.1 miles) if I would skydive from 5,000 feet instead of 10,000 feet. I told him I would be happy to go halfway—I'd take the plane ride up but I wouldn't take the shortcut down.

What I'm getting at is this: You won't be getting good exercise—by that I mean fat-burning exercise—unless it *feels* like exercise. It has to get your heart beating and pores sweating. Only then can you reap all those wonderful benefits I described at the beginning of the chapter.

WHERE'S THE WEIGHT LOSS?

If you're exercising every day and not losing any weight (or, heaven forbid, gaining weight!), it means you're doing something wrong. But it probably has to do with the way you're eating, not the way you're exercising. The following questions will give you a clue as to whether your eating habits are good or bad.

- Do you skip meals and binge on the next?
- Do you use alcohol as a stress and tension release?
- Do you eat while watching television or reading the newspaper?
- Do you eat quickly, hardly chewing your food?
- Do you always finish what's on your plate?
- Do you consume more caffeine daily than you should in order to combat fatigue and increase energy?
- Do you eat dessert every day?
- Do you ignore the calorie content of the foods you eat?
- Do you keep junk food snacks in your desk drawer at work?
- Do you eat and drink to be sociable and not because you're hungry?
- Do you weigh yourself every day instead of once a week?
- Do you try to lose five pounds in a week for a special occasion, and then gain it back?
- Do you snack between meals?
- Do you taste your food while cooking it?
- Do you find yourself always talking about food?
- Do you food shop on an empty stomach?
- Do you keep high-calorie foods in your refrigerator and cupboard?
- Do you eat more cheese and nuts than you realize?
- Do you think you eat like a small bird when perhaps it's more like a vulture?

The answers to all these questions should be no. If you've answered yes to four or more questions, you're due for a little self-improvement in the personal food consumption department. I'd suggest trying to change just two habits weekly for the next ten weeks. By the time you get to the end of the list, you should be losing weight.

If you've passed this test with flying colors then the problem is most likely your exercise program.

Is your exercise really aerobic? Are you doing it every day? You just might need to exercise more. By increasing your daily exercise routine you're bound to get your weight-loss program on the move again.

Charting Your Way

Okay, now, you're on your way. Turn to the charts on the following pages and pick an exercise that's right for you. For the first 30 days you won't be asked to do anything for more than ten minutes.

As I've told you before, whether you walk a mile or jog a mile, you'll be burning approximately 100 calories. But running will give you an edge on cardiovascular benefits. True, we want to accomplish that as well–but, initially, simply covering the distance and doing the exercise is most important.

I believe in the theory of LSD, Long Slow Distance. You need to exercise over a sustained period of time. At first, just concentrate on doing the exercise so that you get committed to it, like it, and feel comfortable with it. If you go too fast, you may develop shortness of breath and all the other nasties that make people drop out–muscle pain, fatigue and the feeling that you are losing any agility you might possess. Trying to speed up your weight loss by running instead of walking isn't going to do you any good if you can't keep it up *every day*. So be patient; start slowly, relax and simply do it daily. You'll build up as you go along. I've designed 90-day programs so you can build up your endurance after your initial 30 days.

Pick a program that will be the easiest to fit into your lifestyle and daily schedule. But, most important, you should try to do the exercise you've picked at the same time every day, preferably in the morning. I like exercise in the morning because it represents the most consistent time of most people's day. In fact, it's a lot like swallowing a natural, long-lasting pep pill. It fills you with plenty of energy and it keeps you going all day long.

FIGHTING THE HUNGRIES

Here is a quick tip to turn off a stomach that's starting to talk back at you. Sit up straight in a chair and pull in your abdominal muscles, holding them as tight as possible for 10 to 20 seconds. Do this five or six times. Your hunger pangs should give up and go away.

WALK
WALK AND JOG

> 10 minutes of walking =
> ½ mile = 50 calories

If exercise is as foreign to you as Sanskrit, I suggest you start out nice and easy–walk. I didn't devise a specific schedule for walking since it's something we all do every day. But you can follow the schedule below, counting all the minutes for walking and jogging as a single walking exercise. Of course, the *faster* you walk, the greater the benefit to your cardiovascular system. And since building a strong heart is good for your health, I expect you to put a little spunk in your walking program. However, I will tell you it won't make any difference in the amount of calories you burn. Speed is unimportant when it comes to burning calories. A mile of walking is 100 calories, just the same as a mile of jogging.

I'm of the belief that if you can walk, you can also jog. So, I devised the schedule below to help turn you from a walker into a jogger. By the middle of Week 4 you'll be jogging a full mile (it should take you about 10 minutes). By the end of Week 12, you'll be getting a full 30 minutes of aerobic exercise.

You don't have to follow this schedule rigidly. Jog more and walk less if you have the energy. If the going gets tough, do more walking than jogging. Just remember: Jog at a pace that's comfortable.

Good luck!

WEEK 1

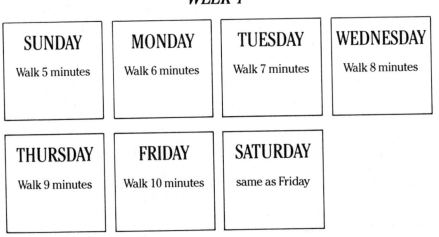

SUNDAY	MONDAY	TUESDAY	WEDNESDAY
Walk 5 minutes	Walk 6 minutes	Walk 7 minutes	Walk 8 minutes

THURSDAY	FRIDAY	SATURDAY
Walk 9 minutes	Walk 10 minutes	same as Friday

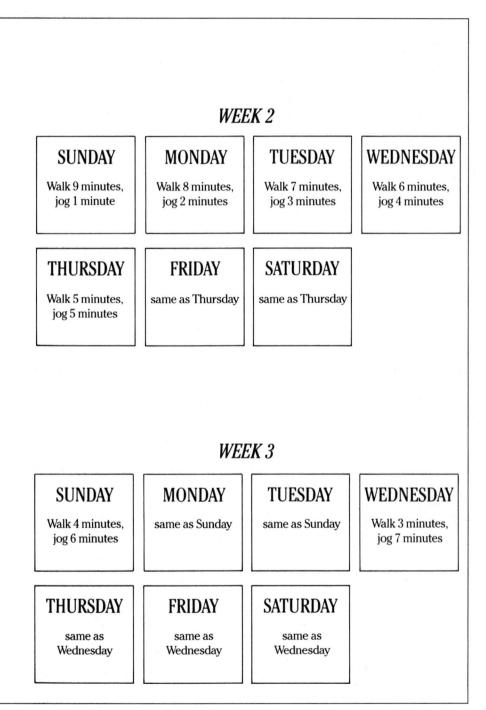

WEEK 2

SUNDAY	MONDAY	TUESDAY	WEDNESDAY
Walk 9 minutes, jog 1 minute	Walk 8 minutes, jog 2 minutes	Walk 7 minutes, jog 3 minutes	Walk 6 minutes, jog 4 minutes

THURSDAY	FRIDAY	SATURDAY
Walk 5 minutes, jog 5 minutes	same as Thursday	same as Thursday

WEEK 3

SUNDAY	MONDAY	TUESDAY	WEDNESDAY
Walk 4 minutes, jog 6 minutes	same as Sunday	same as Sunday	Walk 3 minutes, jog 7 minutes

THURSDAY	FRIDAY	SATURDAY
same as Wednesday	same as Wednesday	same as Wednesday

(Continued)

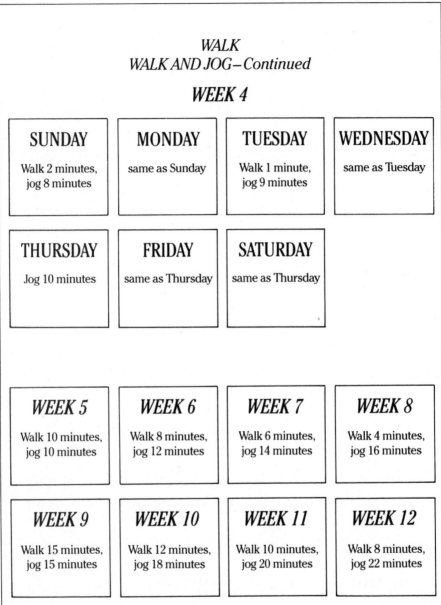

WALK
WALK AND JOG – Continued

WEEK 4

SUNDAY	MONDAY	TUESDAY	WEDNESDAY
Walk 2 minutes, jog 8 minutes	same as Sunday	Walk 1 minute, jog 9 minutes	same as Tuesday

THURSDAY	FRIDAY	SATURDAY	
Jog 10 minutes	same as Thursday	same as Thursday	

WEEK 5	*WEEK 6*	*WEEK 7*	*WEEK 8*
Walk 10 minutes, jog 10 minutes	Walk 8 minutes, jog 12 minutes	Walk 6 minutes, jog 14 minutes	Walk 4 minutes, jog 16 minutes

WEEK 9	*WEEK 10*	*WEEK 11*	*WEEK 12*
Walk 15 minutes, jog 15 minutes	Walk 12 minutes, jog 18 minutes	Walk 10 minutes, jog 20 minutes	Walk 8 minutes, jog 22 minutes

JOGGING PROGRAM

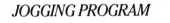

10 minutes = 1 mile = 100 calories

If you want to put a little more effort into your exercise than simply walking, you might want to try this beginner's jogging program. Speed is unimportant in this program. Just make sure you jog at a pace in which you can comfortably talk. This schedule slowly works you up to a great aerobic workout–30 minutes a day of jogging.

WEEK 1	WEEK 2	WEEK 3	WEEK 4
Jog 5 minutes	Jog 6 minutes	Jog 8 minutes	Jog 10 minutes

WEEK 5	WEEK 6	WEEK 7	WEEK 8
Jog 12 minutes	Jog 14 minutes	Jog 16 minutes	Jog 18 minutes

WEEK 9	WEEK 10	WEEK 11	WEEK 12
Jog 20 minutes	Jog 24 minutes	Jog 26 minutes	Jog 30 minutes

BICYCLING

10 minutes = 3 miles = 100 calories

Bicycling is a wonderful conditioning exercise—as long as you're pumping the pedals and not spending too much time coasting downhill. So be honest with yourself. Find a relatively level area or a road with slight hills to ride on so that you can keep your cadence relatively even.

The chart below is for riding outdoors. You're likely to enjoy the exercise much more if you can enjoy some scenery.

Is a stationary bicycle more your style? No problem. Simply add an extra three minutes (about one mile) to each step of the schedule and you will have the same workout. In addition, set the bicycle's tension so that you're feeling slight tension on your quadriceps (the muscle in front of the thigh) and your pulse rate is at 70 percent of maximum (to figure this out, turn to page 48).

Whether you're riding an indoor or outdoor bicycle, make sure the seat is high enough so that your legs are fully extended. If the seat is too low you could end up with knee problems.

WEEK 1

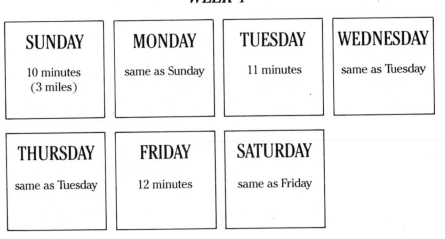

SUNDAY	MONDAY	TUESDAY	WEDNESDAY
10 minutes (3 miles)	same as Sunday	11 minutes	same as Tuesday

THURSDAY	FRIDAY	SATURDAY
same as Tuesday	12 minutes	same as Friday

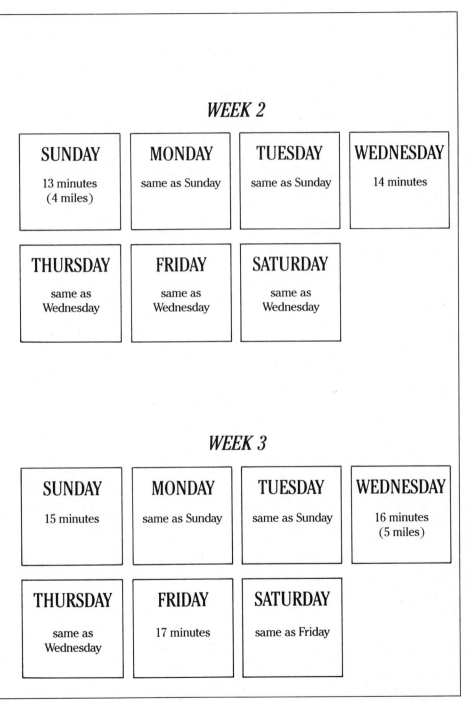

WEEK 2

SUNDAY	MONDAY	TUESDAY	WEDNESDAY
13 minutes (4 miles)	same as Sunday	same as Sunday	14 minutes

THURSDAY	FRIDAY	SATURDAY
same as Wednesday	same as Wednesday	same as Wednesday

WEEK 3

SUNDAY	MONDAY	TUESDAY	WEDNESDAY
15 minutes	same as Sunday	same as Sunday	16 minutes (5 miles)

THURSDAY	FRIDAY	SATURDAY
same as Wednesday	17 minutes	same as Friday

(Continued)

BICYCLING—Continued

WEEK 4

SUNDAY	MONDAY	TUESDAY	WEDNESDAY
18 minutes	same as Sunday	same as Sunday	same as Sunday

THURSDAY	FRIDAY	SATURDAY
19 minutes	same as Thursday	same as Thursday

WEEK 5

SUNDAY	MONDAY	TUESDAY	WEDNESDAY
20 minutes (6 miles)	same as Sunday	same as Sunday	same as Sunday

THURSDAY	FRIDAY	SATURDAY
21 minutes	same as Thursday	same as Thursday

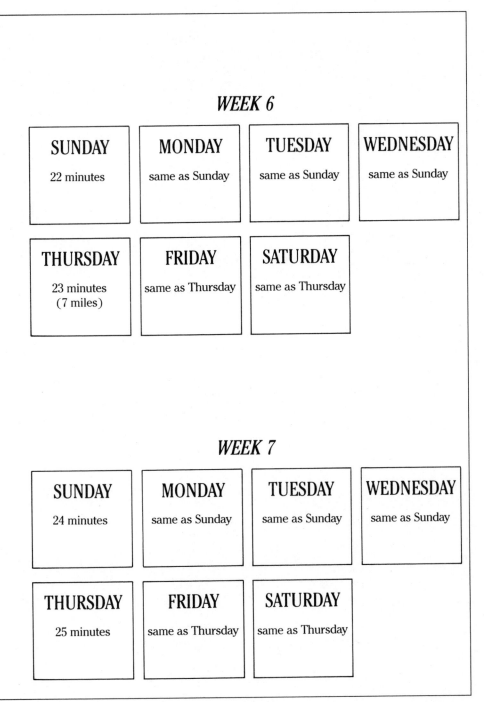

WEEK 6

SUNDAY	MONDAY	TUESDAY	WEDNESDAY
22 minutes	same as Sunday	same as Sunday	same as Sunday

THURSDAY	FRIDAY	SATURDAY
23 minutes (7 miles)	same as Thursday	same as Thursday

WEEK 7

SUNDAY	MONDAY	TUESDAY	WEDNESDAY
24 minutes	same as Sunday	same as Sunday	same as Sunday

THURSDAY	FRIDAY	SATURDAY
25 minutes	same as Thursday	same as Thursday

(Continued)

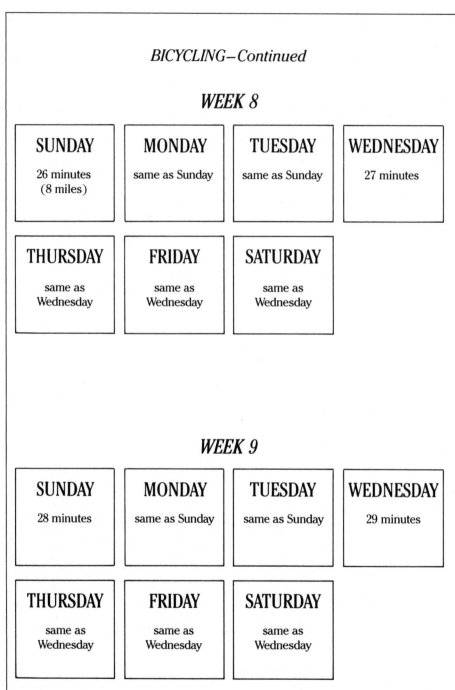

BICYCLING—Continued

WEEK 8

SUNDAY	MONDAY	TUESDAY	WEDNESDAY
26 minutes (8 miles)	same as Sunday	same as Sunday	27 minutes

THURSDAY	FRIDAY	SATURDAY
same as Wednesday	same as Wednesday	same as Wednesday

WEEK 9

SUNDAY	MONDAY	TUESDAY	WEDNESDAY
28 minutes	same as Sunday	same as Sunday	29 minutes

THURSDAY	FRIDAY	SATURDAY
same as Wednesday	same as Wednesday	same as Wednesday

WEEK 10

SUNDAY 30 minutes (9 miles)	**MONDAY** same as Sunday	**TUESDAY** same as Sunday	**WEDNESDAY** 31 minutes
THURSDAY same as Wednesday	**FRIDAY** 32 minutes	**SATURDAY** same as Friday	

WEEK 11

SUNDAY 33 minutes (10 miles)	**MONDAY** same as Sunday	**TUESDAY** 34 minutes	**WEDNESDAY** same as Tuesday
THURSDAY same as Tuesday	**FRIDAY** 35 minutes	**SATURDAY** same as Friday	

(Continued)

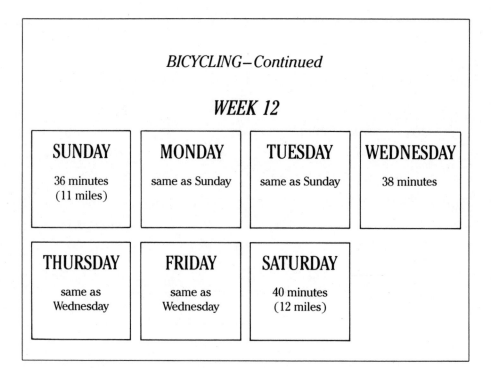

BICYCLING—Continued

WEEK 12

SUNDAY	MONDAY	TUESDAY	WEDNESDAY
36 minutes (11 miles)	same as Sunday	same as Sunday	38 minutes

THURSDAY	FRIDAY	SATURDAY
same as Wednesday	same as Wednesday	40 minutes (12 miles)

SWIMMING

> 10–12 minutes = 400 meters (¼ mile)
> = 100 calories

If you're a water bug, you'll find swimming a wonderful way to get in your daily exercise quotient. This schedule, however, assumes you haven't been swimming in quite some time. It starts you out at a modest 5 lengths and gradually works you up to one mile—64 lengths—by the end of Week 12.

If you're swimming now, but not on a daily basis, you'll want to start where it's comfortable for you and progress at your own speed. Just make sure you do it every day.

This schedule is based on swimming freestyle in a 25-meter pool at a moderate speed—10 to 12 minutes for every 400 meters, or ¼ mile. If the length of your pool is different, adjust the time accordingly. Swimming faster, of course, will burn more calories. Swimming breaststroke or butterfly will also burn more calories.

WEEK 1

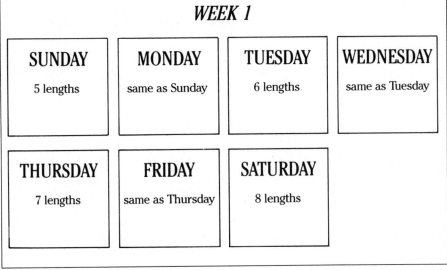

SUNDAY	MONDAY	TUESDAY	WEDNESDAY
5 lengths	same as Sunday	6 lengths	same as Tuesday

THURSDAY	FRIDAY	SATURDAY
7 lengths	same as Thursday	8 lengths

(Continued)

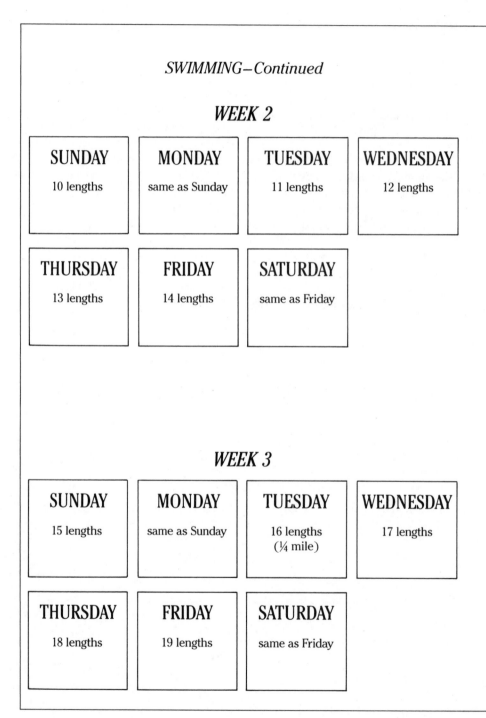

SWIMMING—Continued

WEEK 2

SUNDAY	MONDAY	TUESDAY	WEDNESDAY
10 lengths	same as Sunday	11 lengths	12 lengths

THURSDAY	FRIDAY	SATURDAY
13 lengths	14 lengths	same as Friday

WEEK 3

SUNDAY	MONDAY	TUESDAY	WEDNESDAY
15 lengths	same as Sunday	16 lengths (¼ mile)	17 lengths

THURSDAY	FRIDAY	SATURDAY
18 lengths	19 lengths	same as Friday

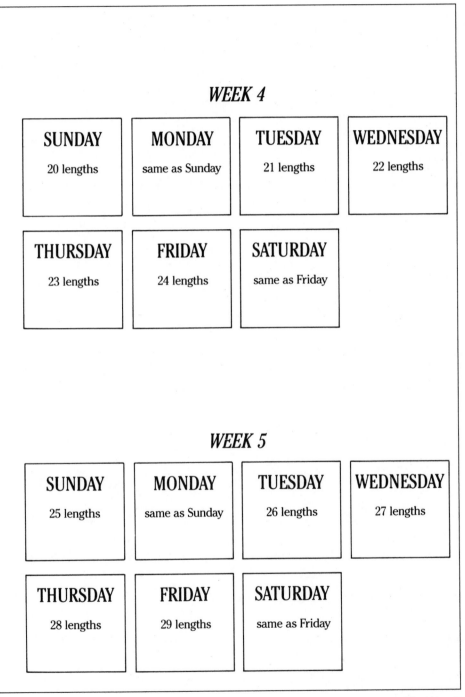

WEEK 4

SUNDAY	MONDAY	TUESDAY	WEDNESDAY
20 lengths	same as Sunday	21 lengths	22 lengths

THURSDAY	FRIDAY	SATURDAY
23 lengths	24 lengths	same as Friday

WEEK 5

SUNDAY	MONDAY	TUESDAY	WEDNESDAY
25 lengths	same as Sunday	26 lengths	27 lengths

THURSDAY	FRIDAY	SATURDAY
28 lengths	29 lengths	same as Friday

(Continued)

SWIMMING—Continued

WEEK 6

SUNDAY	MONDAY	TUESDAY	WEDNESDAY
30 lengths	same as Sunday	31 lengths	32 lengths (½ mile)

THURSDAY	FRIDAY	SATURDAY
33 lengths	34 lengths	same as Friday

WEEK 7

SUNDAY	MONDAY	TUESDAY	WEDNESDAY
35 lengths	same as Sunday	36 lengths	37 lengths

THURSDAY	FRIDAY	SATURDAY
38 lengths	39 lengths	same as Friday

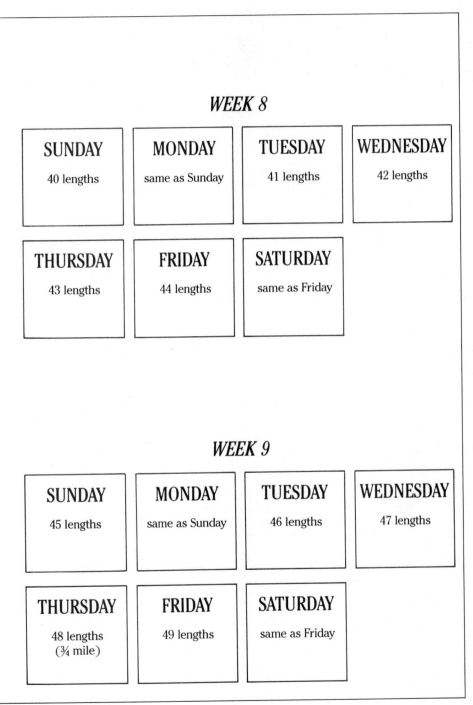

WEEK 8

SUNDAY	MONDAY	TUESDAY	WEDNESDAY
40 lengths	same as Sunday	41 lengths	42 lengths

THURSDAY	FRIDAY	SATURDAY
43 lengths	44 lengths	same as Friday

WEEK 9

SUNDAY	MONDAY	TUESDAY	WEDNESDAY
45 lengths	same as Sunday	46 lengths	47 lengths

THURSDAY	FRIDAY	SATURDAY
48 lengths (¾ mile)	49 lengths	same as Friday

(Continued)

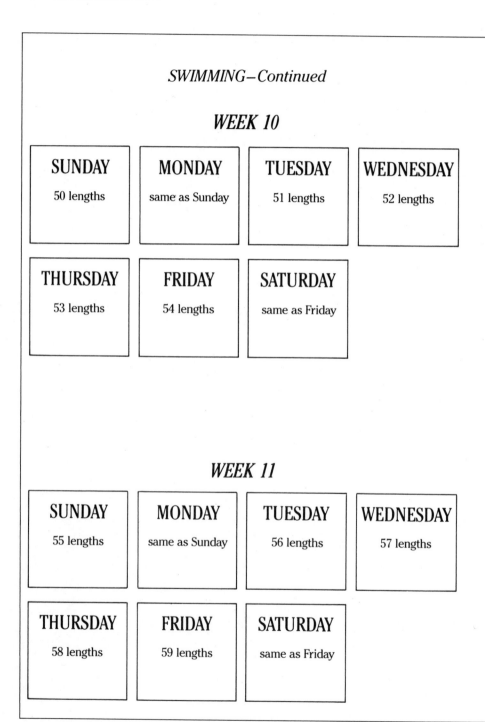

SWIMMING—Continued

WEEK 10

SUNDAY	MONDAY	TUESDAY	WEDNESDAY
50 lengths	same as Sunday	51 lengths	52 lengths

THURSDAY	FRIDAY	SATURDAY
53 lengths	54 lengths	same as Friday

WEEK 11

SUNDAY	MONDAY	TUESDAY	WEDNESDAY
55 lengths	same as Sunday	56 lengths	57 lengths

THURSDAY	FRIDAY	SATURDAY
58 lengths	59 lengths	same as Friday

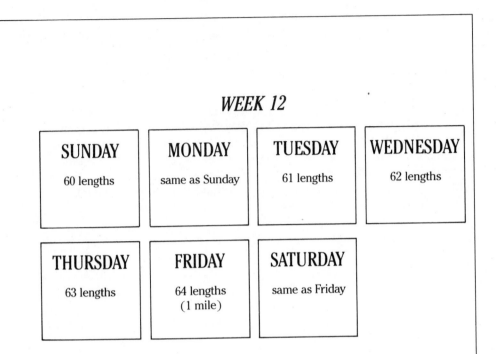

WEEK 12

SUNDAY	**MONDAY**
60 lengths	same as Sunday

TUESDAY	**WEDNESDAY**
61 lengths	62 lengths

THURSDAY	**FRIDAY**
63 lengths	64 lengths (1 mile)

SATURDAY
same as Friday

MINITRAMPOLINE OR REBOUNDER

10 minutes = 75 calories

Many people are under the impression that jumping on a minitrampoline or rebounder provides the same aerobic conditioning and burns the same amount of calories as jogging. This simply is not true. However, I don't dismiss it as an exercise. If you can bear the monotony of bouncing about in a confined space for an extended length of time, the schedule below should provide you with a good and easy-to-follow workout. You should always land one foot at a time.

WEEK 1	WEEK 2	WEEK 3	WEEK 4
10 minutes	10 minutes	10 minutes	10 minutes

WEEK 5	WEEK 6	WEEK 7	WEEK 8
11 minutes	11 minutes	12 minutes	12 minutes

WEEK 9	WEEK 10	WEEK 11	WEEK 12
13 minutes	13 minutes	14 minutes	15 minutes

JUMPING ROPE

10 minutes = 700 steps = 150 calories

Jumping rope is a great exercise, but if you haven't done it in 10 or 20 years (or even longer) don't expect to get back in the swing of things too easily. It may look like a breeze, but five minutes of jumping rope for a novice exerciser can seem like a very long time!

You can jump with two feet together or one foot at a time, but a step counts as each contact with the floor. The calories burned will depend upon the intensity and speed of your jumping.

Do not jump on a surface that's too hard (jumping rope is really tough on the knees and lower legs), and make sure you wear a pair of sneakers or other soft-soled shoes.

WEEK 1

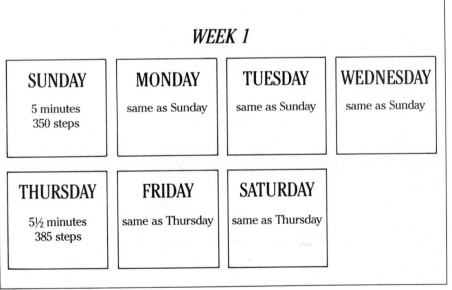

SUNDAY	MONDAY	TUESDAY	WEDNESDAY
5 minutes 350 steps	same as Sunday	same as Sunday	same as Sunday

THURSDAY	FRIDAY	SATURDAY
5½ minutes 385 steps	same as Thursday	same as Thursday

(Continued)

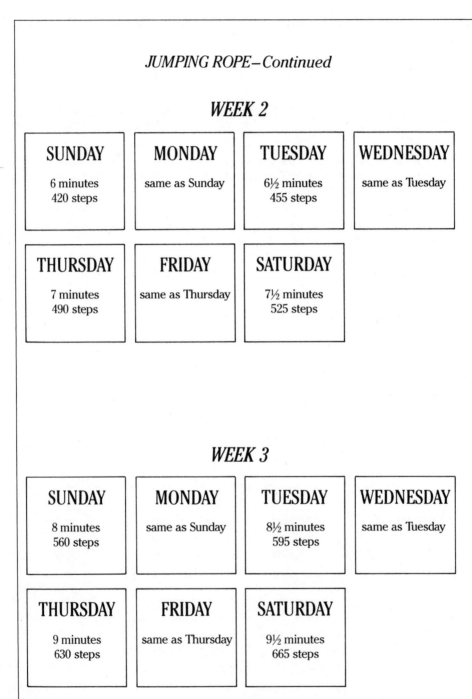

JUMPING ROPE–Continued

WEEK 2

SUNDAY	MONDAY	TUESDAY	WEDNESDAY
6 minutes 420 steps	same as Sunday	6½ minutes 455 steps	same as Tuesday

THURSDAY	FRIDAY	SATURDAY
7 minutes 490 steps	same as Thursday	7½ minutes 525 steps

WEEK 3

SUNDAY	MONDAY	TUESDAY	WEDNESDAY
8 minutes 560 steps	same as Sunday	8½ minutes 595 steps	same as Tuesday

THURSDAY	FRIDAY	SATURDAY
9 minutes 630 steps	same as Thursday	9½ minutes 665 steps

WEEK 4

SUNDAY 10 minutes 700 steps	**MONDAY** same as Sunday	**TUESDAY** 10½ minutes 735 steps	**WEDNESDAY** same as Tuesday
THURSDAY 11 minutes 770 steps	**FRIDAY** same as Thursday	**SATURDAY** 11½ minutes 805 steps	

WEEK 5

SUNDAY 12 minutes 840 steps	**MONDAY** same as Sunday	**TUESDAY** 12½ minutes 875 steps	**WEDNESDAY** same as Tuesday
THURSDAY 13 minutes 910 steps	**FRIDAY** same as Thursday	**SATURDAY** 13½ minutes 945 steps	

(Continued)

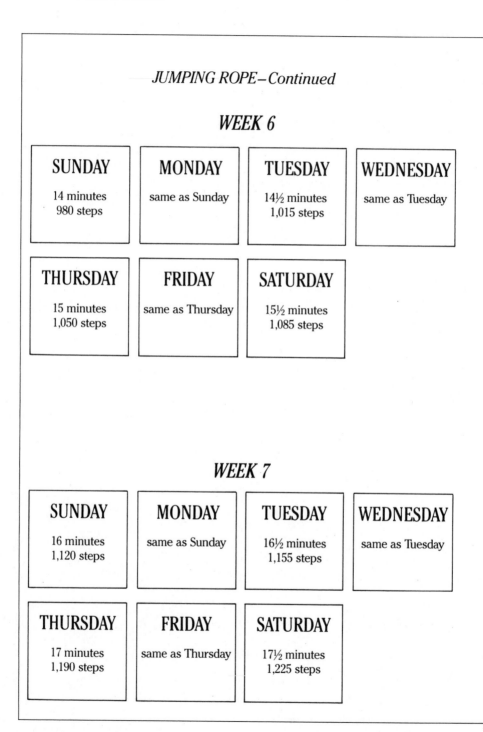

JUMPING ROPE—Continued

WEEK 6

SUNDAY	MONDAY	TUESDAY	WEDNESDAY
14 minutes 980 steps	same as Sunday	14½ minutes 1,015 steps	same as Tuesday

THURSDAY	FRIDAY	SATURDAY
15 minutes 1,050 steps	same as Thursday	15½ minutes 1,085 steps

WEEK 7

SUNDAY	MONDAY	TUESDAY	WEDNESDAY
16 minutes 1,120 steps	same as Sunday	16½ minutes 1,155 steps	same as Tuesday

THURSDAY	FRIDAY	SATURDAY
17 minutes 1,190 steps	same as Thursday	17½ minutes 1,225 steps

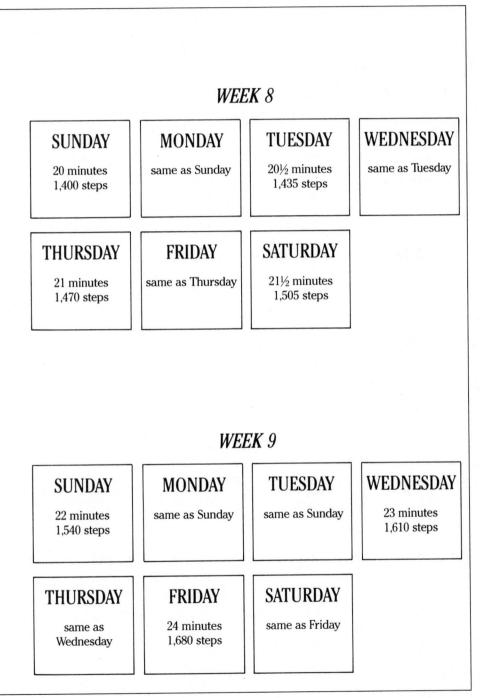

WEEK 8

SUNDAY	MONDAY	TUESDAY	WEDNESDAY
20 minutes 1,400 steps	same as Sunday	20½ minutes 1,435 steps	same as Tuesday

THURSDAY	FRIDAY	SATURDAY
21 minutes 1,470 steps	same as Thursday	21½ minutes 1,505 steps

WEEK 9

SUNDAY	MONDAY	TUESDAY	WEDNESDAY
22 minutes 1,540 steps	same as Sunday	same as Sunday	23 minutes 1,610 steps

THURSDAY	FRIDAY	SATURDAY
same as Wednesday	24 minutes 1,680 steps	same as Friday

(Continued)

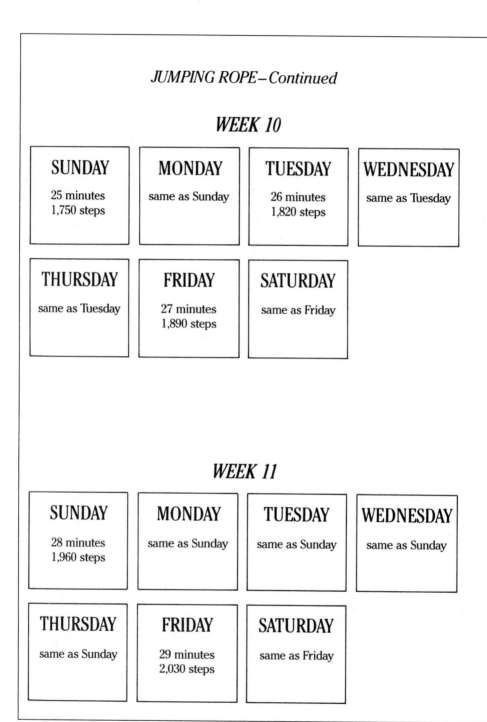

JUMPING ROPE–Continued

WEEK 10

SUNDAY	MONDAY	TUESDAY	WEDNESDAY
25 minutes 1,750 steps	same as Sunday	26 minutes 1,820 steps	same as Tuesday

THURSDAY	FRIDAY	SATURDAY
same as Tuesday	27 minutes 1,890 steps	same as Friday

WEEK 11

SUNDAY	MONDAY	TUESDAY	WEDNESDAY
28 minutes 1,960 steps	same as Sunday	same as Sunday	same as Sunday

THURSDAY	FRIDAY	SATURDAY
same as Sunday	29 minutes 2,030 steps	same as Friday

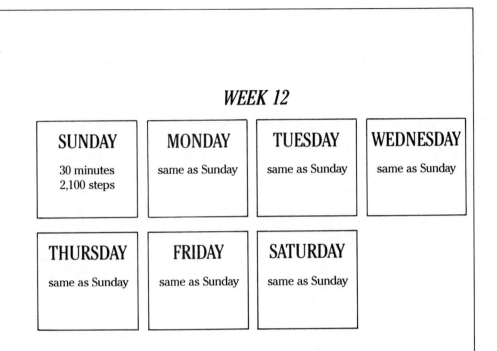

WEEK 12

SUNDAY 30 minutes 2,100 steps	**MONDAY** same as Sunday	**TUESDAY** same as Sunday	**WEDNESDAY** same as Sunday
THURSDAY same as Sunday	**FRIDAY** same as Sunday	**SATURDAY** same as Sunday	

AEROBIC DANCING

10 minutes = 30 to 50 calories

This one is tough to accurately gauge, because much depends on the class (or to be more precise, the teacher) and the way you perform in it.

Thirty minutes of a class does not mean 30 minutes of aerobics. Every class contains 5 to 10 minutes of warm-up and cool-down stretching, strengthening and toning exercises. (If it doesn't, get out of it and find one that does.) So, even though the schedule below lists a 30-minute class to start out with, you can count on getting about 10 minutes of real aerobic exercise.

Aerobic tapes, however, are an altogether different story. Most tapes are almost *all* aerobics. So, if you're using a tape, start out with 10 to 15 minutes for the first four weeks, increase to 20 minutes the fifth week and work up until you're at 30 minutes of aerobics by Week 12. And remember to warm up and cool down with these workouts, even if such exercises aren't included in the tape.

Make sure you monitor your pulse rate so that it doesn't get too high. Some classes can be pretty tough on a novice, so remember to always exercise on the side of caution. If you feel that it's getting to be too much for you, slow down, almost to a stop if need be. Don't worry about what everyone else is doing.

WEEK 1 30-minute class	*WEEK 2* 30-minute class	*WEEK 3* 30-minute class	*WEEK 4* 30-minute class
WEEK 5 40-minute class	*WEEK 6* 40-minute class	*WEEK 7* 40-minute class	*WEEK 8* 40-minute class
WEEK 9 50-minute class	*WEEK 10* 50-minute class	*WEEK 11* 50-minute class	*WEEK 12* 60-minute class

ROWING

10 minutes = 175 calories

Of course, I mean a rowing *machine*, not meandering about in a canoe. And it's one hard exercise. So hard, in fact, I don't expect you to start out with ten minutes a day. Instead, I've made ten minutes your 30-day goal!

When it comes to an aerobic workout, rowing ranks right up there with the best. The number of calories you burn, of course, will depend on the intensity of the exercise and the number of strokes you are able to complete in a minute.

Rowing, by the way, is a great exercise for someone with orthopedic problems because it doesn't put much stress on the joints.

WEEK 1	WEEK 2	WEEK 3	WEEK 4
5 minutes a day	7 minutes a day	8 minutes a day	10 minutes a day
WEEK 5	WEEK 6	WEEK 7	WEEK 8
12 minutes a day	15 minutes a day	18 minutes a day	20 minutes a day
WEEK 9	WEEK 10	WEEK 11	WEEK 12
23 minutes a day	25 minutes a day	28 minutes a day	30 minutes a day

STAIR CLIMBING

| 10 minutes = 25 flights = 200 calories |

Stair climbing—and I mean going up *only*—is very strenuous and should be done as a routine exercise only by healthy individuals and with approval from a physician. One flight of stairs is considered ten steps. You should be able to climb between two and three flights every minute.

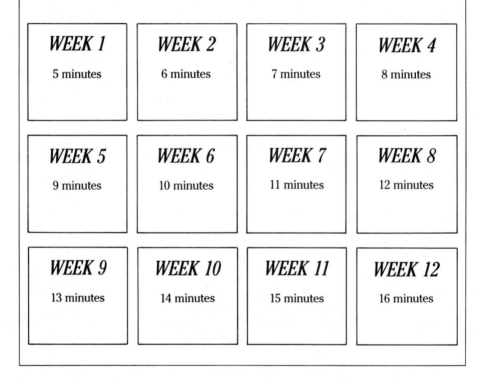

WEEK 1 5 minutes	**WEEK 2** 6 minutes	**WEEK 3** 7 minutes	**WEEK 4** 8 minutes
WEEK 5 9 minutes	**WEEK 6** 10 minutes	**WEEK 7** 11 minutes	**WEEK 8** 12 minutes
WEEK 9 13 minutes	**WEEK 10** 14 minutes	**WEEK 11** 15 minutes	**WEEK 12** 16 minutes

SPORTS COMBO

Looking for competition? If you like to participate in recreational sports such as racquetball, handball, tennis or basketball, you can alternate them with your ten-minutes-a-day solo aerobic exercise routine. However, since some recreational sports don't provide the heart-conditioning or calorie-burning capacity of more aerobic-type exercise, you'll have to plan on spending more time at them. For example, 10 minutes of jogging equals 40 to 60 minutes of amateur tennis playing.

If you're going to substitute a recreational sport for your aerobic exercise, just make sure that the sport is physically demanding. Sorry, but no miniature golf!

Below is a sample program that incorporates five different types of exercise. You can follow this one or make up your own.

WEEK 1

SUNDAY	MONDAY	TUESDAY	WEDNESDAY
Tennis 40 to 60 minutes	Racquetball* 30 minutes	Jumping rope† 5 minutes	Tennis 40 to 60 minutes

THURSDAY	FRIDAY	SATURDAY
Jog or walk 10 minutes	Racquetball 30 minutes	Stair climbing 8 minutes

Handball may be substituted for racquetball.
†Jumping rope and stair climbing may be interchanged.

(Continued)

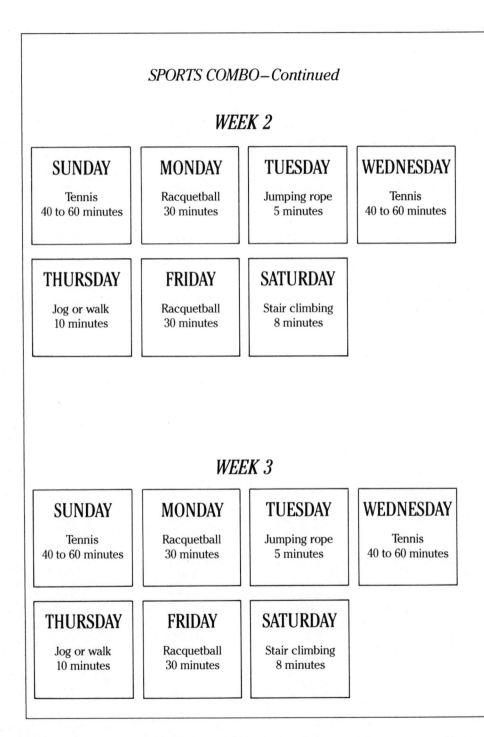

SPORTS COMBO—Continued

WEEK 2

SUNDAY	MONDAY	TUESDAY	WEDNESDAY
Tennis 40 to 60 minutes	Racquetball 30 minutes	Jumping rope 5 minutes	Tennis 40 to 60 minutes

THURSDAY	FRIDAY	SATURDAY
Jog or walk 10 minutes	Racquetball 30 minutes	Stair climbing 8 minutes

WEEK 3

SUNDAY	MONDAY	TUESDAY	WEDNESDAY
Tennis 40 to 60 minutes	Racquetball 30 minutes	Jumping rope 5 minutes	Tennis 40 to 60 minutes

THURSDAY	FRIDAY	SATURDAY
Jog or walk 10 minutes	Racquetball 30 minutes	Stair climbing 8 minutes

WEEK 4

SUNDAY	MONDAY	TUESDAY	WEDNESDAY
Tennis 40 to 60 minutes	Racquetball 30 minutes	Jumping rope 5 minutes	Tennis 40 to 60 minutes

THURSDAY	FRIDAY	SATURDAY
Jog or walk 10 minutes	Racquetball 30 minutes	Stair climbing 8 minutes

WEEK 5

SUNDAY	MONDAY	TUESDAY	WEDNESDAY
Tennis 60 minutes	Racquetball 45 minutes	Jumping rope 8 minutes	Tennis 60 minutes

THURSDAY	FRIDAY	SATURDAY
Jog or walk 15 minutes	Racquetball 45 minutes	Stair climbing 10 minutes

(Continued)

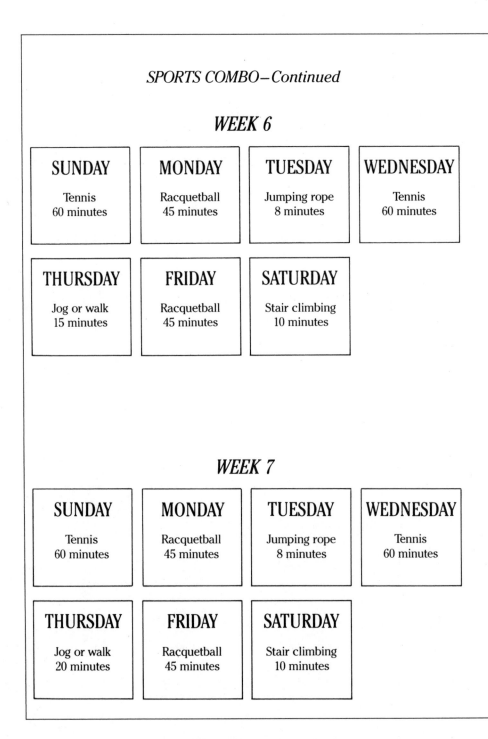

SPORTS COMBO—Continued

WEEK 6

SUNDAY	MONDAY	TUESDAY	WEDNESDAY
Tennis 60 minutes	Racquetball 45 minutes	Jumping rope 8 minutes	Tennis 60 minutes

THURSDAY	FRIDAY	SATURDAY
Jog or walk 15 minutes	Racquetball 45 minutes	Stair climbing 10 minutes

WEEK 7

SUNDAY	MONDAY	TUESDAY	WEDNESDAY
Tennis 60 minutes	Racquetball 45 minutes	Jumping rope 8 minutes	Tennis 60 minutes

THURSDAY	FRIDAY	SATURDAY
Jog or walk 20 minutes	Racquetball 45 minutes	Stair climbing 10 minutes

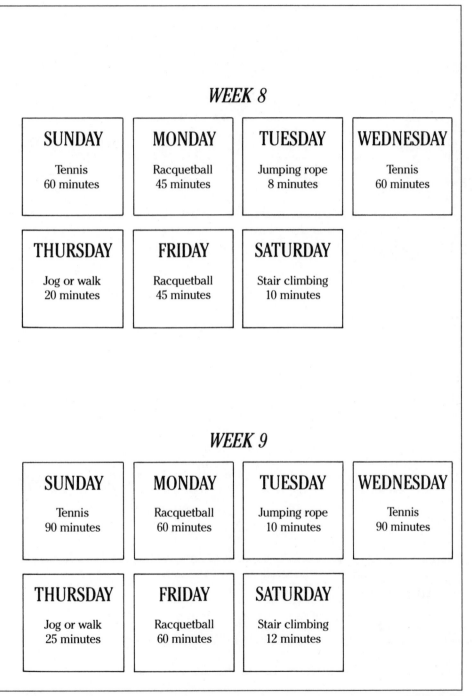

WEEK 8

SUNDAY	MONDAY	TUESDAY	WEDNESDAY
Tennis 60 minutes	Racquetball 45 minutes	Jumping rope 8 minutes	Tennis 60 minutes

THURSDAY	FRIDAY	SATURDAY
Jog or walk 20 minutes	Racquetball 45 minutes	Stair climbing 10 minutes

WEEK 9

SUNDAY	MONDAY	TUESDAY	WEDNESDAY
Tennis 90 minutes	Racquetball 60 minutes	Jumping rope 10 minutes	Tennis 90 minutes

THURSDAY	FRIDAY	SATURDAY
Jog or walk 25 minutes	Racquetball 60 minutes	Stair climbing 12 minutes

(Continued)

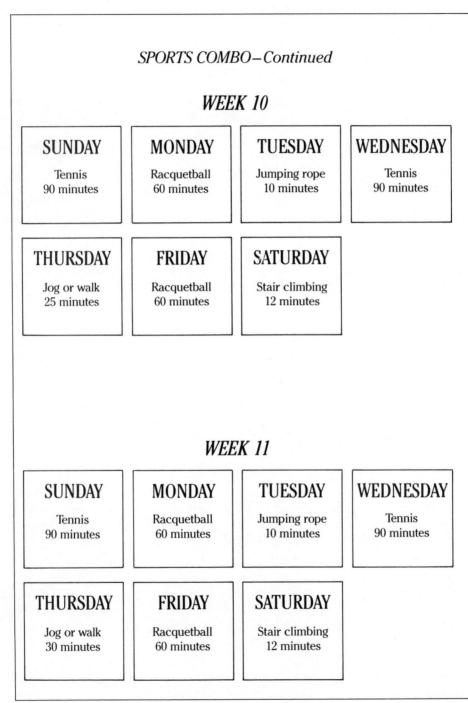

SPORTS COMBO–Continued

WEEK 10

SUNDAY	MONDAY	TUESDAY	WEDNESDAY
Tennis 90 minutes	Racquetball 60 minutes	Jumping rope 10 minutes	Tennis 90 minutes

THURSDAY	FRIDAY	SATURDAY
Jog or walk 25 minutes	Racquetball 60 minutes	Stair climbing 12 minutes

WEEK 11

SUNDAY	MONDAY	TUESDAY	WEDNESDAY
Tennis 90 minutes	Racquetball 60 minutes	Jumping rope 10 minutes	Tennis 90 minutes

THURSDAY	FRIDAY	SATURDAY
Jog or walk 30 minutes	Racquetball 60 minutes	Stair climbing 12 minutes

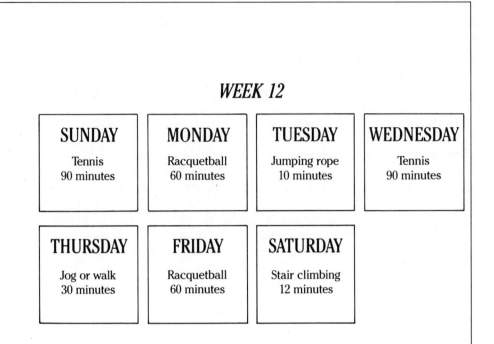

WEEK 12

SUNDAY	MONDAY	TUESDAY	WEDNESDAY
Tennis 90 minutes	Racquetball 60 minutes	Jumping rope 10 minutes	Tennis 90 minutes

THURSDAY	FRIDAY	SATURDAY
Jog or walk 30 minutes	Racquetball 60 minutes	Stair climbing 12 minutes

THE VARIETY ACT

Does jogging or walking day in and day out sound boring to you? In fact, if doing the same kind of *any* type of exercise day after day is more than you're willing to endure, I've got the program for you. It combines four different types of aerobic exercise, but no two days in a row are the same!

In this program you're going to count distance, not minutes (after all, you are looking for something different), although you can figure you'll be spending around 10 minutes at each exercise every day for the first four weeks and building up to 30 minutes by the time you reach Week 12.

Here are a few reminders:

Walk and jog at a speed that is comfortable and at which you can carry on a conversation.

Swimming lengths are based on a 25-meter pool. If your pool is a different size, compensate by varying the number of lengths accordingly.

Bicyling (whether it's indoor or out) should be strenuous enough that you feel tension in your quadriceps, the large muscle in front of the thigh.

WEEK 1

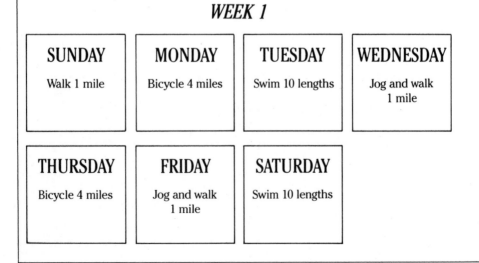

SUNDAY	MONDAY	TUESDAY	WEDNESDAY
Walk 1 mile	Bicycle 4 miles	Swim 10 lengths	Jog and walk 1 mile

THURSDAY	FRIDAY	SATURDAY
Bicycle 4 miles	Jog and walk 1 mile	Swim 10 lengths

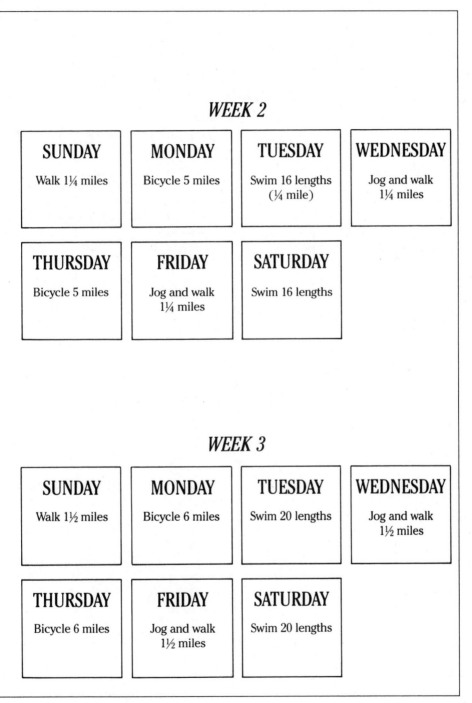

WEEK 2

SUNDAY	MONDAY	TUESDAY	WEDNESDAY
Walk 1¼ miles	Bicycle 5 miles	Swim 16 lengths (¼ mile)	Jog and walk 1¼ miles

THURSDAY	FRIDAY	SATURDAY
Bicycle 5 miles	Jog and walk 1¼ miles	Swim 16 lengths

WEEK 3

SUNDAY	MONDAY	TUESDAY	WEDNESDAY
Walk 1½ miles	Bicycle 6 miles	Swim 20 lengths	Jog and walk 1½ miles

THURSDAY	FRIDAY	SATURDAY
Bicycle 6 miles	Jog and walk 1½ miles	Swim 20 lengths

(Continued)

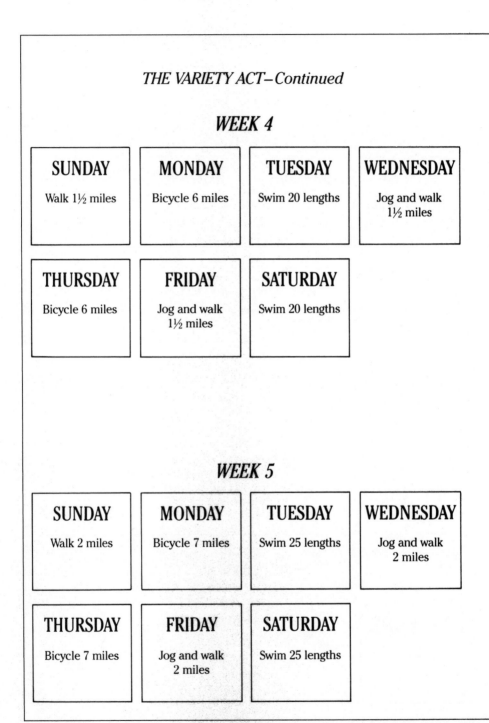

THE VARIETY ACT–Continued

WEEK 4

SUNDAY	MONDAY	TUESDAY	WEDNESDAY
Walk 1½ miles	Bicycle 6 miles	Swim 20 lengths	Jog and walk 1½ miles

THURSDAY	FRIDAY	SATURDAY
Bicycle 6 miles	Jog and walk 1½ miles	Swim 20 lengths

WEEK 5

SUNDAY	MONDAY	TUESDAY	WEDNESDAY
Walk 2 miles	Bicycle 7 miles	Swim 25 lengths	Jog and walk 2 miles

THURSDAY	FRIDAY	SATURDAY
Bicycle 7 miles	Jog and walk 2 miles	Swim 25 lengths

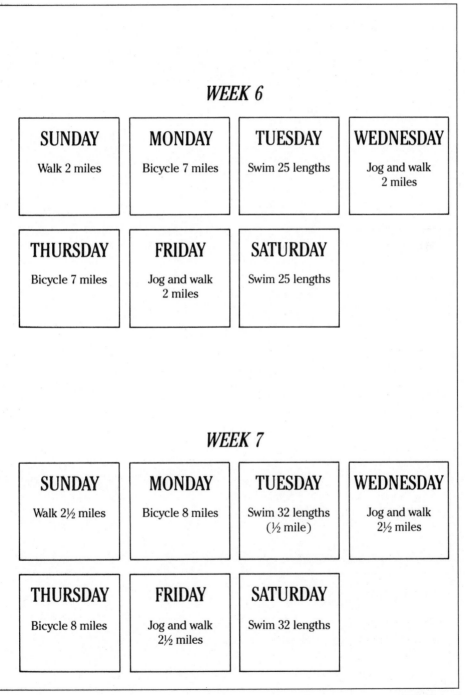

WEEK 6

SUNDAY	MONDAY	TUESDAY	WEDNESDAY
Walk 2 miles	Bicycle 7 miles	Swim 25 lengths	Jog and walk 2 miles

THURSDAY	FRIDAY	SATURDAY
Bicycle 7 miles	Jog and walk 2 miles	Swim 25 lengths

WEEK 7

SUNDAY	MONDAY	TUESDAY	WEDNESDAY
Walk 2½ miles	Bicycle 8 miles	Swim 32 lengths (½ mile)	Jog and walk 2½ miles

THURSDAY	FRIDAY	SATURDAY
Bicycle 8 miles	Jog and walk 2½ miles	Swim 32 lengths

(Continued)

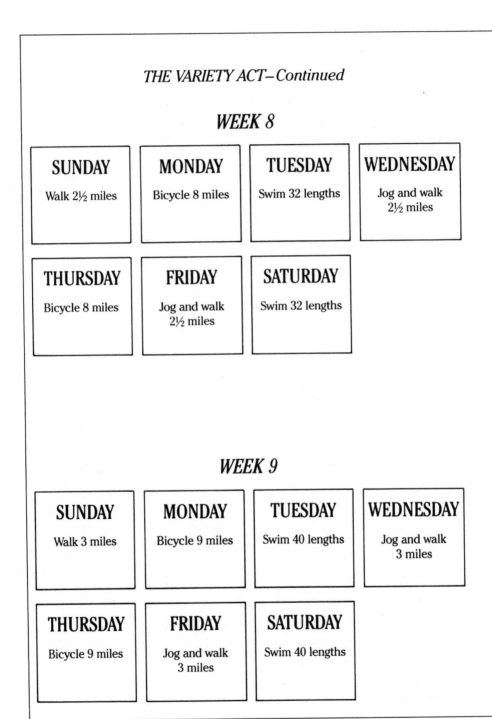

THE VARIETY ACT—*Continued*

WEEK 8

SUNDAY	MONDAY	TUESDAY	WEDNESDAY
Walk 2½ miles	Bicycle 8 miles	Swim 32 lengths	Jog and walk 2½ miles

THURSDAY	FRIDAY	SATURDAY
Bicycle 8 miles	Jog and walk 2½ miles	Swim 32 lengths

WEEK 9

SUNDAY	MONDAY	TUESDAY	WEDNESDAY
Walk 3 miles	Bicycle 9 miles	Swim 40 lengths	Jog and walk 3 miles

THURSDAY	FRIDAY	SATURDAY
Bicycle 9 miles	Jog and walk 3 miles	Swim 40 lengths

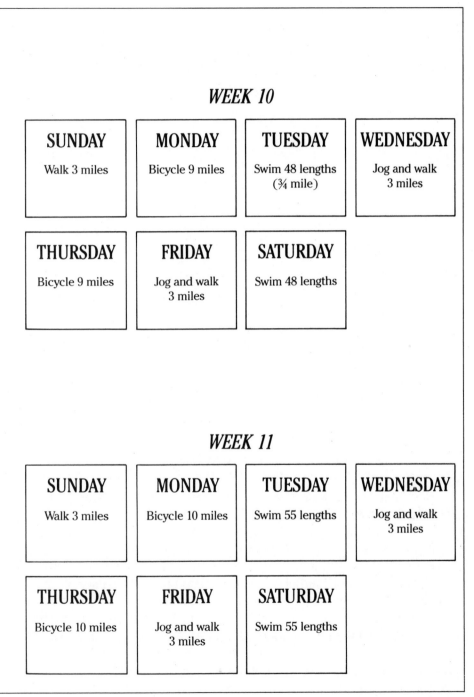

WEEK 10

SUNDAY	MONDAY	TUESDAY	WEDNESDAY
Walk 3 miles	Bicycle 9 miles	Swim 48 lengths (¾ mile)	Jog and walk 3 miles

THURSDAY	FRIDAY	SATURDAY
Bicycle 9 miles	Jog and walk 3 miles	Swim 48 lengths

WEEK 11

SUNDAY	MONDAY	TUESDAY	WEDNESDAY
Walk 3 miles	Bicycle 10 miles	Swim 55 lengths	Jog and walk 3 miles

THURSDAY	FRIDAY	SATURDAY
Bicycle 10 miles	Jog and walk 3 miles	Swim 55 lengths

(Continued)

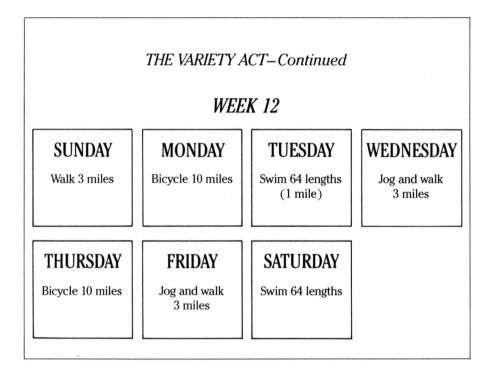

THE VARIETY ACT—Continued

WEEK 12

SUNDAY	MONDAY	TUESDAY	WEDNESDAY
Walk 3 miles	Bicycle 10 miles	Swim 64 lengths (1 mile)	Jog and walk 3 miles

THURSDAY	FRIDAY	SATURDAY
Bicycle 10 miles	Jog and walk 3 miles	Swim 64 lengths

Exercise Level for Starting Programs

Now that you've looked at the programs, perhaps you're thinking, "Hey, the first two weeks will be a breeze. I already exercise at Week 3 level." Wrong again! If that's the case, I want you to *start* at Week 3.

If you can start with Week 3 or even Week 6 because you're in good shape, then all the better for you. Start with a higher level of fitness and simply increase accordingly. For instance, if you'd prefer to exercise for 20 to 30 minutes a day in the beginning then, by all means, do it. But you must do it every day in order to receive the full benefit, and the minimal addictive dose, of the Mollen Method. Just because you're doing twice the exercise, doesn't mean you can do it every other day. Or, if you feel after two days of Week 2 that you can comfortably advance to Week 3, simply increase your exercise based upon your ability.

If you've been playing a recreational sport and want to stick with it alone, then plan on playing it every day. But remember, you'll have to play it every day for close to an hour. If that's impossible, substitute another activity such as walking or bicycling on non-playing days.

I understand that not everyone has a lot of time to spare for exercise and that's one of the reasons I list the minimal amount of time you should spend doing each exercise. If time is a problem, simply pick one that requires less. For example, if you're rushed in the first week, jump rope for five to eight minutes and you're done for the day. Everyone has ten minutes to spare in their day. That's all it takes. More time and less effort? Try walking a mile. You've got to find the time to do it. It's a priority!

Building Momentum

Want to speed up your progress on the Mollen Method? Here are a few things you can do for yourself to boost your energy output.

If you're already involved in a sport you like–one that requires some length of time, like basketball, racquetball, golf, tennis or even bowling–I'd like you to increase your playing time. For example, if you shoot baskets with the boys two days a week after work, start making it three. If you play racquetball one night a week for an hour, start playing two nights. If you

---

MISSED A DAY? THE QUICK MAKE-UP METHOD

Everybody has excuses–a marathon airplane trip; a stomach virus that won't let you get up, let alone get out to exercise; a dinner party that went into the wee hours of the morning; a snow storm that left a barricade at your door. Missing a day of exercise is forgivable once in a while–as long as you make it up.

Now this doesn't mean that I'm revoking my edict that in order to make the Mollen Method successful you must exercise every day. What I'm telling you is that if you *do* miss a day for some reason (and you'd better have a good excuse), you can make it up. How? Simply double up on your exercise routine the following day–ten minutes in the morning and another ten in the evening.

However, it's best not to depend on this too often, for before you know it, you'll be trying to make up all your exercise in just one full-blown effort.

have one bowling night out a week, make it two. (Of course, you'll have to forgo the tradition of "going out for a few beers afterwards.")

But I want you to do these things in addition to, and not in lieu of, your ten-minute aerobic workout. The truth is, unless you're a Larry Bird, a Chris Evert Lloyd or a class A racquetball or handball player, these exercises aren't allowing you to sustain your heart rate at its optimum aerobic level long enough to qualify as a really good *aerobic* workout. And most people don't play at championship levels. But many sports are beneficial nevertheless, and they do keep you active. And activity burns a lot more calories than passivity.

How many calories you actually burn (no matter what the charts tell you) depends on how hard you play the game. If you're just "batting the ball around the court," you're not getting nearly the workout (and calorie-burning benefits) of someone whose opponent is really giving him or her a rough time. If you are a good player and decide to double your playing time each week, you're sure to notice some difference in your weight. And even your game.

The idea is to stay extremely active when following the Mollen Method. And I'm not just talking exercise. Being active could mean anything, whether it's involvement with community projects, accompanying the kids on a field trip, or taking up dog grooming. I want you to become a doer, not a sitter.

By maintaining a higher level of activity you won't have time to think about food. How many diets have you been on during which you've done nothing but live from one meal to the next, with only work, sleep and maybe a little activity in between? Turn that into a lot of activity—exercise combined with meaningful and fun things to do—and you won't have time to listen to your stomach growl.

The Stairway to Fitness

There's another thing I'd like you to do as you initiate yourself in your new life of exercise. Forget elevators and escalators were ever invented. I want you to climb the stairs every opportunity you get.

Stair climbing is an excellent way to condition your heart. As an added bonus, it burns many calories—some 1,200 per hour—which is more than swimming or even running.

Unfortunately, stair climbing is hard work and you won't be doing it an hour at a shot. But you can do it every chance you get.

Better yet, you might want to make it your ten-minute-a-day exercise. I, for one, would be proud of you if you did. The benefits to your health would be tremendous. A study in Finland a few years back showed that men who climbed about 25 flights of stairs during the course of a day lost a significant amount of weight after only 12 weeks. That may sound like a lot of stairs, but let's think about it for a moment. Everyone encounters stairs every day. How often do you avoid them by taking the elevator? If you live in a two-story house, how often do you avoid a little extra exertion by using the first floor powder room instead of going upstairs? A little bit of stair climbing can measure up to a lot of exercise in the long run.

If you work in a high-rise office building, why not start a stair-climbing club? Consider your building a mountain you want to conquer. Climb each day, keeping tabs on how many feet each person can manage. The winner is the one who ascends first. For instance, if you plan to climb Mount Everest at approximately 30,000 feet, that would be equivalent to approximately 60,000 steps. Since each flight of stairs is approximately 10 steps it would require 6,000 flights to reach the top.

However, as with any exercise a certain amount of caution must be used. Since stair climbing puts a tremendous load on your heart, I recommend you go slowly and monitor your pulse rate every ten flights to make sure it's not getting too high. If you experience dizziness or lightheadedness you're probably going too fast. Slow down and simply take it one step at a time.

Excuses, Excuses

"I don't have time to exercise." If I've heard this excuse once from my patients, I've heard it a thousand times. Lack of time seems to be the universal excuse for avoiding exercise. In fact, lack of time even supersedes the excuse that exercising is boring.

My reply is this: You've got to make the time to exercise because it's important to your health. For instance, if you have small children, either hire a baby-sitter for an hour daily or find a friend who also has small children and take turns watching each other's children. An alternative solution when you have small children is to buy a stationary bicycle and ride while they nap.

Another common excuse that people use to avoid exercise is that they go to work early in the morning and get home late. Obviously, these people are going to have to change their priorities in order to incorporate exercise

A BIT ABOUT BODY BUILDING

There are various ways to develop muscular strength and endurance. One way is through exercises that cause muscles to contract, such as isotonic and isometric exercises.

Isotonic exercises involve muscular contractions with joint movement. Certain weight-training exercises—either with free weights or Nautilus-type equipment—are isotonic exercises. Isometric exercises cause muscles to contract without producing any movement in a joint or limb. An abdominal contraction is an isometric exercise. Another type of isometric exercise requires resistance, such as grasping your hands together and applying a steady tension, hand against hand. This resistance helps develop muscle tone and strength.

Isotonics are generally considered better exercises for developing muscles than isometrics, since they enhance the flexibility and elasticity of the muscles as well as develop strength and endurance. However, isotonics require equipment (free weights, Nautilus, Universal Gym and Cam II are popular) and a place in which to use them, such as a health club, gym or spa. If this type of program interests you, find a reputable place with a qualified instructor who can set you up in an individual program.

Isometrics are much more convenient because they require no equipment or basic skills. The nicest thing about them is that they can be done almost anywhere and at any time.

in their life. My suggestion is to go home at night and before eating dinner get on a stationary bicycle for 10 to 15 minutes to unwind from the day. An alternative to this would be simply to jump rope for 5 minutes before going to work in the morning.

Most people can find a fitness program they can work into their day if they look hard enough. The truth is that ten minutes a day devoted to exercise is not too much for anyone. I find that the morning is the easiest time of day to exercise and be consistent about it. It's easy to make exercise habit forming when you do it first thing, just like brushing your teeth. However, some people may find that skipping lunch and substituting exercise is the best program for them. If you exercise instead of eating lunch, have a couple pieces of fruit to satisfy your hunger throughout the afternoon. Others find that exercising after work is the best way to unwind.

The "absence of time" syndrome can also be related to how effectively you're utilizing the rest of your day. If you honestly can't find the time for exercise, you should consider taking a time-management course. It'll show you how to improve the efficiency of your overall workday. I'm sure you'll be able to find room for exercise.

A final reason often used as an excuse for not exercising is family commitments: "My kids need my attention after work," or "My wife gets angry when I'm running instead of mowing the lawn." My solution for these types of problems is to simply involve your family in an exercise program with you. It could mean joining a health club, bicycling together or walking several miles after dinner. Such togetherness also makes motivation come more naturally. And once that addictive dose grabs hold, excuses will be no more, even when you're away from home.

If She Can, You Can

If you're reading this and thinking you're too fat, too old, too out of shape or too tired to start the Mollen Method, then read the story of my patient, Sally.

When she was nine years old, Sally was thrown from a horse. She was in a coma for three weeks and, when she became conscious, she couldn't walk or talk. It took her eight weeks to learn how to talk and get back on her feet, although she was left with a leg that drags. She depended on a leg brace to help her get around. As you can tell from her story that follows, Sally was a real trooper. She wasn't going to let her disability stand in the way of her desire to become a doer, not a sitter.

I'll let her tell the story, in her own words:

"Because of the accident, I had no muscle tone at all. I had to start out from scratch in building muscles, strength and endurance.

"The first race I was in was the 1982 Phoenix 10K. A friend gave me an entry blank and it quoted Dr. Mollen as saying, 'Run, jog, walk or crawl, but join us.' I decided to enter.

"At that point I wasn't embarrassed, but I was insecure about walking and limping among all those veteran runners. I told myself, well, it is not going to get any easier.

"I got to the track and walked through the crowd and people were urging me on. It was great. I had on a plastic brace. Because I didn't have running shoes, I wore my work shoes.

"I did about two miles in that race. But nobody put me down, they cheered me on. I decided I wanted to do better. So I wrote to Dr. Mollen asking for advice for runners who have partial paralysis. He answered, saying he'd see me free of charge.

"The first thing he did was put me on a weight-loss program. The extra weight would be too hard on my leg and the brace if I were to run, he said. He gave me incentive. I lost 15 pounds.

"I was ready for my first full-fledged 10K race about three months later. I was quickly left in back of the pack, but I didn't mind. All I wanted to do was finish. When I approached the finish line, I heard my name over the loudspeaker. They even held up the award ceremony to wait for me. When I crossed the finish line, all of a sudden three thousand runners were cheering. It was exhilarating.

"I just know that if it wasn't for Dr. Mollen's program, today I'd be 240 pounds and doing nothing, nothing at all.

"But can you imagine it? There were three thousand people cheering for me. Of all people, me. I can't believe it."

So, what's your excuse? If you still think you're too fat, too old, too out of shape or too tired, then think of Sally. I won't buy your excuses. You know you can do it and so does Sally.

Still not convinced? Then listen to this story from one of my other patients, Frank:

"There's an old saying that inside every heavy person there's a thin person trying to get out. I should know, because I was large enough to be hiding several of those thin people. At 425 pounds, life was no longer fun. In fact, I knew it was gong to come to an abrupt end if I didn't allow that thin person inside me to emerge from those thick walls of fat. Surely we would both die. Then along comes this doctor who tells me to exercise. Good grief, I could barely *move*!

"Finding clothes to fit was a real problem and one that I found very embarrassing. I wore 58-inch-waist pants. As far as restaurants went, I had to eliminate all those that had only booths. I was simply too big to fit into them. And some chairs were even becoming a problem.

"Can you imagine going to someone's house for the first time and having them tell you where to sit, then never being invited back because you are so heavy they are afraid you'll break their furniture?

"My car was another problem. In order to be able to drive I had to have the front seat back as far as it would go and the steering wheel tilted up in the highest position. It's not as if I was trying to squeeze into a compact car because I drove one of the biggest cars on the road—a Lincoln Mark V. While sitting in the car, my stomach pressed against the steering wheel and my head pushed against the roof. When you are as heavy as I was you have a lot of extra padding to sit on which makes you appear taller when seated.

"Even with all the problems, I still didn't care. I just kept eating and eating and eating. I was becoming more and more unhappy. I was slowly but surely killing myself with food.

"So I decided to take Dr. Mollen's advice and exercise. He started me on a walking program. At first I hated walking, but after several weeks I started to enjoy it.

"A year later, I had lost 195 pounds. Then I started running and the weight seemed to come off faster. Running has been an essential part of my weight-loss program. Six months after I began running, I was down to 195 and I was ready for my first 10K race. I ran it in 49:44. I kept running in races. A year later I completed my first triathlon—a 1.2-mile swim, followed by 56 miles on a bicycle, followed by a 13-mile run. It took me six and a half hours to finish."

Frank completed the triathlon in 1983, an unbelievable accomplishment considering where he had started. I even envied him. Why? He beat me by 30 minutes and was standing at the finish line with a diet soft drink in his hand waiting for me. With a rather sardonic smile on his face he asked, "What took you so long, Doc?"

Take a Cue from Glen Campbell

Still not convinced that the Mollen Method is for you? How about a testimonal from Glen Campbell, the country and western singer. Glen has been my patient for several years, but I was having a hard time trying to convince him what a good time exercise could be. I kidded him that "By the Time I Get to Exercise" could be the title of his next hit song. It seemed to be one of his most popular excuses. Motivation finally hit after his marriage.

Now Glen doesn't live religiously by the Mollen Method, but he does take the exercise part seriously. He spends *at least* ten minutes each day exercising and admits "I feel great."

Most of Glen's friends and family agree that he looks and feels better than he has in the last ten years.

So there it is. The first part of the Mollen Method, all neatly set out for you. All you have to do is select the exercise that seems to suit you and your circumstances best, reset your alarm clock so that you get up a little earlier each day, and you're in business.

The payoff? Weight loss. Total well-being.

Make the commitment and start today. Now. In fact, it's not a bad idea to go ahead and take a walk right this minute. When you come back, read the next chapter about food and diet.

Chapter 5

EATING – THE MOLLEN WAY

I love to eat. Ask anyone who's ever had dinner with me and they'll tell you that I can eat an entire loaf of bread at one sitting. Not only do I *always* eat dessert, but I often go back for seconds, and sometimes even thirds. And dining in a gourmet restaurant is one of the things I enjoy most.

Yes, I'm what you'd probably call one of the lucky ones. I can munch away on all the foods I love without gaining an ounce. I weigh 155 pounds today and I'll weigh 155 pounds tomorrow. I can bank on it. But luck really has nothing to do with it. There is a very logical reason why I can eat what I eat without gaining weight.

Naturally, the fact that I exercise two hours a day has a lot to do with it. (You've already learned—and should be convinced—that exercise is crucial to any weight control plan because it burns calories and increases metabolism.) But that's only *part* of it.

The rest has to do with what I eat. Or, more precisely, what I *don't* eat.

Sure, I can polish off a loaf of bread—but you'll never see me touch it with butter or margarine. Yes, I love to eat dessert—but the desserts I eat are always fresh fruits (strawberries are my favorite) and I always eat them plain. New York's finest chef can serve me an elegant Dover sole—but I'll always politely push the sauce aside, even if it is described as "light and nonfattening."

You see, what I don't eat is fat—the fat that's 99 proof in butter, the fat that forces you to let out your belt a notch after you eat a rich dessert or dine on meat and sauces laden with cream, cheese or butter.

And the foods that I *love* are vegetables and fruits and the variety of things that can be made from wonderful grains. Sure I can eat them to my heart's content. Why not! They're wonderfully nutritious, which means they're good for me. They're low in calories, so I don't have to worry about counting them. But most important of all, the foods I love are low in fat.

And that, in a nutshell, is the key to my diet—low fat.

Doing It My Way

Now don't jump to conclusions and think that you can eat yourself into oblivion as long as you don't eat fatty foods. It doesn't quite work that way. Sure, I can put away a lot of food—now. But there was a time in my life when I couldn't. When I was getting out of medical school I was 25 pounds overweight and couldn't manage to run a mile without gasping for air. My favorite foods were Philadelphia cheese steaks and pizzas with extra cheese. I loved whole milk and would drink it by the quart. My cholesterol was high and so were my triglycerides. Then I started to notice all the people in the hospital where I worked who had just passed age 40—the age I am now—looking overweight, out of shape and older than their years. I didn't want the same thing to happen to me.

I knew exercise and proper diet were important but I wasn't sure how to make them work for me. So I reopened my nutrition books with a new interest in mind—me. I knew I had to lower my fat consumption to lower my perilous cholesterol and triglyceride counts. I knew the right thing to do was to increase my intake of fruits and vegetables—complex carbohydrates—to give me the energy I lacked. But I didn't know how to do it in a style that I would like. Living on nothing but greens and apples didn't sound all that appealing. I knew I needed protein, too, but at first I didn't realize how little I needed. I found out that protein actually works better for you when it's combined with complex carbohydrates. So I eliminated the high-protein foods which contain large amounts of fat, like meat (in fact, I haven't touched it since), and took up foods that combined protein *and* carbohydrates, like grains and starchy vegetables, which I love.

I built a program around all these foods—fruits, vegetables, cereals, rice, potatoes, beans. I took up jogging and body building. In three months I had dropped my extra weight, my cholesterol and triglyceride counts were normal, my energy was high and I had adopted a way of eating that I truly enjoyed.

That was more than 15 years ago. Today I look and feel better than I ever have in my life. I'm in peak condition. And a body in peak condition burns calories most efficiently. That's why I don't have a weight problem

SENSIBLE WEIGHT-LOSS PRINCIPLES

- Set reasonable goals for yourself. You did not gain the weight overnight and you will not lose the weight overnight.
- Avoid weighing yourself daily because your body weight can fluctuate daily. Instead, weigh yourself once a week.
- Tell your family and friends you are trying to lose weight and ask for their support.
- Avoid talking about food—you'll only make yourself unhappy.
- Do not shop when you are hungry—this leads to buying unnecessary food.
- Be aware of the caloric content of all the foods you eat. Cut calories from recipes:
    Replace sour cream with yogurt.
    Replace whole milk with skim milk.
    Replace high-fat cheese with low-fat cheese.
- Do not taste food as you are cooking; if necessary, enlist a "taster."
- Eat food in one area, the kitchen or dining room, not the living room or bedroom.
- Do not watch television or listen to the radio while eating.
- After you have portioned out your food, immediately put leftovers away to avoid tempting yourself.
- A smaller plate will make your meal appear larger.
- Eat the lower calorie foods first.
- Eat and chew slowly. Studies show a direct relationship between rate of eating and total caloric consumption of a meal.
- Eating light (not creamy) soup at a meal may help decrease the amount of food eaten as well as slow the rate at which it is eaten.
- Do not eat simply because everyone else is eating.
- Do not use food as a reward.
- Eat a large salad before going to a party. If you don't feel hungry, you won't be tempted to nibble on party food.
- If you live alone, or with other dieters, do not keep high-calorie foods in the house.
- Hunger pangs usually last ten minutes and will go away without your giving in to them. Go for a walk or exercise to get your mind off of them until they pass.
- Activity will increase calories burned.
- Activity will help suppress your appetite.

any more. My body's only 8 percent fat, meaning I have plenty of muscle and muscle burns calories faster than fat. At 8 percent body fat I can burn the same amount of calories a lot faster than someone who is 25 percent body fat—even if we're both sitting around doing nothing.

Can the same thing happen to you? Of course, *if* you follow the Mollen Method. But like me, you'll have to start at the beginning–by shaving fat, from your body and your diet.

Why Less Fat?

Take a look in the mirror. I'll bet there's plenty that's pleasant to look at–like an attractive face, beautiful hair, maybe even a boastful waistline. Now take a look at the unpleasant parts. You may have a thin waist, but do you have thighs that are almost as big? Do your buttocks detract from your figure? Does your stomach hang over your belt instead of sitting snugly within? You know what to call that excess flesh–fat. In men, fat has a tendency to collect in the abdominal area; it's *the* popular place for fat cells to congregate. In women, they're generally more widespread, collecting in the buttocks, hips, thighs, breasts. How do these areas get so flabby? From eating too much fat. Fat on the menu turns into fat in the body. It's as simple as that. Eliminate that fat–or reduce it dramatically–and you'll also notice a dramatic change in the way you look. And the way you feel.

The reason there are so many fat Americans (36 million are considered overweight) is because Americans as a whole eat too much fat. People in the United States consume 42 percent of their calories from fat–more than twice the amount my patients learn to eat. Sound amazing? Not when you consider how much fat there is in the foods that we eat, and not when you consider how easily it is hidden.

Fat isn't all that easy to identify. Sure, just about everyone knows that the likes of butter, oil and lard are almost pure fat. But only one-third of the fat we get in our diet comes from such "recognizable" fat. The other two-thirds is hidden. Foods such as eggs, cheese, variety crackers, fast foods, processed meats, olives and nuts are all high in fat. They don't look like fat–like the fat we can readily recognize as butter or lard–but it's there. Put a flavored cracker on a paper towel and pick it up a few hours later. It'll leave a greasy spot behind–fat. Take a nice creamy cheese and set it out for a few hours at room temperature. You'll find it swimming in fat. Nuts, olives. Where do you think peanut oil and olive oil come from? Their namesakes, of course.

We love our red meat juicy and tender so we eat meats that are well marbled or, put another way, "fattened up." The higher the marbling, the higher the grade, the higher the price, the higher the fat. No wonder people are so confused!

The Fat Attack

Why do fats work against you and not for you? For one thing, fats are the highest source of calories available. Every ounce of fat contains more than twice the calories you'll find in an ounce of protein or an ounce of carbohydrates. One tablespoon of butter, for example, is 102 calories. You can eat it in just moments and it won't do a thing to satisfy your appetite. But for the same number of calories you can eat a whole apple. It takes a lot of chewing to get that apple to disappear, and it'll keep you feeling full for hours.

Fat works against you in another way: It takes longer to digest than other foods. When it comes to burning fuel, your body much prefers carbohydrates. And carbohydrates are slow burners (that's why you feel satisfied longer), so the fat has to wait around for its turn to get into digestive action. On idle, it only makes you feel sluggish. Often the fat isn't called on at all for energy use (which can happen when you eat too much or don't burn enough calories through exercise), and it takes a permanent rest—right in those cushy fat cells. When it comes to seeking tenants, fat cells always have their "vacancy" signs glowing.

But there is a way to put those fat cells out of business. By cutting back on fat you'll slow down the amount of fat that is being deposited in those spots you consider so unattractive. And when your body turns to fat for fuel, it'll start taking it from the places where it's plentiful, like your stomach, thighs or buttocks. And it goes without saying that cutting back on fats can be nothing but good for your health. Lower fat naturally means a lower level of cholesterol and triglycerides and a decreased risk of heart disease.

So, on the Mollen Method you'll reduce fat to 20 percent.

What you'll be giving up in fat, you'll be making up in other foods that are good for you—carbohydrates and, to a lesser degree, protein. To best explain how these foods will work *for* you (as opposed to fat which works *against* you), we'll have to take a quick course in nutrition.

The Two Faces of Carbohydrates

Carbohydrates come in two forms: simple, which you should eat sparingly, and complex, which you should eat abundantly. Simple carbohydrates are simple sugars which are found in such things as sugar, honey, jellies and other sweets. Because they are simple in chemical form, our bodies break them down very rapidly, causing our blood sugar to rise quickly and just as quickly take a dip. We don't want this to happen because it can lead to fatigue, moodiness and even worse—hunger.

Oh, you'll eat simple carbohydrates on the Mollen Method but in very small doses, like a dab of honey on your bread or a bit of sugar in your dessert. Just enough to give you taste, and always combined with other good things so you won't suffer the roller-coaster ill effects. So when I tell you to eat plenty of carbohydrates, don't reach for a box of jelly doughnuts. That's not what I'm talking about.

What I want you to eat are the good-guy carbohydrates, the ones called complex, found in foods like whole grain breads, high-fiber cereals (not the sugary varieties), vegetables and fruits. These are the foods that are kind to our bodies. They break down in our system slowly, causing sugar to trickle into our bloodstreams, giving us plenty of energy and a satisfied feeling that will last for hours. This is the same kind of food that gives athletes the stamina to go "the extra mile." (It'll give you the stamina to go your distance, too.) And because our bodies use carbohydrates for fuel first, we don't have to worry about them sitting in our system looking for somewhere to go—like a fat cell.

So, on the Mollen Method you'll increase complex carbohydrates to 65 percent.

Protein—Good in Small Doses

Think of protein food and the first thing that most likely comes to mind is a thick slab of steak. How many times have you looked at that steak and said, "Now that's got plenty of protein!" You bet it does. Too much. The truth is, the body doesn't need all that protein. Americans consume far too much protein, four to eight times more than they actually need. And that's not good.

Protein is very similar in chemical makeup to carbohydrates except it contains an extra element—nitrogen. Too much nitrogen creates nasty by-products in our bodies, which must be detoxified by the liver and excreted through the kidneys. Too much protein makes our organs work too hard. The fact that our kidneys must work so hard also means that we stand a chance of losing vital minerals—minerals we need for muscle function and bone strength—through urine. As a result we feel zapped of energy—we can't make that "extra mile."

Our bodies need protein to build and repair tissue. That's protein's main function. As a fuel it's very inefficient, just like fat. It's the body's *last* choice for fuel. Protein that isn't used winds up as fat.

One way to get your protein is from meat, poultry, fish and eggs. These are well-known high-protein foods. The problem is that they give you *a lot* of protein, so you should eat them in small portions.

However, there's a much better way to get your protein—from foods that contain both carbohydrates and protein. This way you get a wider choice of food and more of it. These are foods like low-fat dairy products, grains and starchy vegetables (such as beans, corn, rice and lentils). This is actually the preferred kind of protein. Why? Because in the presence of carbohydrates protein works more efficiently in the body. Carbohydrates contain the vitamins and minerals needed to properly metabolize the protein for use where it is needed—for building and repairing body tissue.

So, on the Mollen Method, you'll limit your protein to 15 percent.

The Diet—Getting Started

Now that I've given you the basics, it's time to get down to the particulars. But before I get started I'd like to explain a little about the 20-percent-fat, 65-percent-carbohydrate and 15-percent-protein ratio.

First of all, when I'm referring to percentages, I'm not referring to the weight of the food, I'm referring to the percentage of fat, carbohydrate or protein from the calories in the food. For example, if you're on a 1,000-calorie-a-day diet and you're permitted 20 percent fat, it means that 200 of those 1,000 calories will be from fat.

Of course, it's bad enough having to count calories, but it's short of impossible to try to figure out the percentage of certain types of food you're allowed to eat each day. But, don't worry, you won't have to do it. I've already done it for you. On pages 158–99 you'll find a 30-day diet plan in each of three caloric categories (1,000, 1,500 and 2,000 calories) already programmed for the Mollen Method.

You don't like being told what you have to eat at each meal? No problem there. All you need do is follow the Mollen Method Menu Plan on pages 125–51 and you can devise your own daily menus. And there's no need to go out and buy a calorie chart. As long as you abide by the serving sizes, stay within the serving limitations in the column "Servings per Day," and only eat the foods allowed, you'll automatically fall within your chosen caloric range.

The second thing I want to tell you is that this 20-65-15 ratio is your *goal*—the type of eating you'll aim to follow for the rest of your life. It's easy. It's practical. But you won't start eating this way until the fourth week of the diet. Before that, it's a little more restrictive. You'll be getting less fat and more carbohydrates (protein, by the way, always remains the same).

I'm sure you remember in the beginning of the book I told you that the Mollen Method is a diet that gets easier as it goes along. (In fact, it may be the reason you bought this book!) Now's the time for me to explain what that means to you.

THE CALORIE COUNT THAT'S RIGHT FOR YOU

The number of calories an individual needs each day to maintain or lose weight is impossible to accurately gauge. So much depends on body size, age, activity, exercise and individual metabolism.

What all this means is that one 124-pound, 30-year-old woman could maintain her weight quite well on 2,000 calories a day while the same style of eating could make another 124-pound, 30-year-old woman gain weight.

Knowing this doesn't help you at all in deciding which diet plan you should follow. Will it be the 1,000-, 1,500- or 2,000-calorie plan?

To help you out, here's a rule of thumb which you can use as a guideline: First determine the weight you want to be. If you're a man, multiply that weight by 15. If you're a woman, multiply that weight by 12. For example, a 170-pound man who wished to be 150 pounds would multiply 150 by 15.

$$150 \times 15 = 2,250$$

He would follow the 2,000-calorie-a-day plan.

A 115-pound woman who wanted to get down to 100 pounds would multiply 100 pounds times 12.

$$100 \times 12 = 1,200$$

She would follow the 1,000-calorie-a-day program.

This equation is based on the premise that you're a person of moderate activity—the *least* that is expected of you on the Mollen Method. If you aren't this active (and be honest), then your daily caloric needs would be even less.

The only thing I want to stress is to be practical in selecting a calorie plan. You should not go on a caloric restriction so severe that it could cause you to become weak and out of sorts. For example, a 200-pound man who wants to lose 50 pounds and plans to exercise 20 minutes a day should not, by any means, go on the 1,000-calorie program. It's much too low. He should follow the 2,000-calorie plan. On the other hand, a 130-pound woman who wants to lose 20 pounds can't expect to do it by eating 2,000 calories a day. For her, the 1,000-calorie-a-day plan would be the right one.

The proper calorie count should make you lose weight steadily, but gradually.

Week 1

The Week 1 menus are the toughest to follow. That's because you'll be limited to only 5 percent fat. But it won't seem that strict when you realize how many different foods you'll actually be allowed to eat on the diet. I've added plenty of variety to keep your taste buds stimulated. As you can probably guess, a restriction to 5 percent fat means you'll be getting plenty of carbohydrates this week–80 percent.

Go ahead, take a look at the menus right now for Week 1. Cereals, fruit juices, milkshakes, an egg (yes, only one this week), fish, a toasted cheese sandwich, potatoes, spaghetti, rice, bread, even apple butter–they're all there; and that's on the 1,000-calorie-a-day diet, the most limited one of all! Of course, you'll eat plenty of fruits and vegetables, and in an appetizing way.

What you won't find are foods heavy in fat, like butter or margarine. You'll learn to eat your bread dry (like I do) or with a little apple butter or fruit preserves. You'll drink skim milk only, eat cheeses that are low in fat and make salad dressings without oil (fat).

Take a look at those menus again. Sure, you can live on that for a week. After all, the beginning of a diet is always easy–it's when you have the most incentive.

To add to your incentive, you'll discover immediate weight loss. Weight comes off fast the first week. And think of all the wonderful things such a healthy diet will be doing for your body!

Think of Week 1 as a week of purification, in which your arteries will gain freedom from fat, your intestines will gain the help of high-fiber foods to smooth along the job of digestion and elimination, your energy stores will gain the rich shot of vitamins and minerals they need to get you rolling on the Mollen Method. If you have problems, just give me a call. I'll be there to give you a pep talk.

Week 2

It's getting better already. This is the week you'll double your fat intake. Double! You're up to 10 percent now. This week you'll experiment a little more in the kitchen by making some of the low-fat desserts and other dishes developed for the Mollen Method. You'll try Pears in Wine and Fruit Blintzes. Sound good, don't they? You'll also sample a low-fat coleslaw and vegetable dishes with a little zip in them. You'll even have French toast for breakfast. We're talking about the real thing, not some insipid "diet" variety!

This is the week you'll reintroduce poultry into your life and, if you wish, alcohol (there's more on this later). Oh, yes, I almost forgot. You'll find a dab of margarine here and there. Whole fat (as I like to call it) is back in your life already.

Week 3

Eating is getting back to normal and you're still losing weight. And feeling wonderful, too. What could be better?

How about some tortillas, a few croutons in your salad, a peanut butter and banana sandwich, chili (made with turkey, not beef)? You'll find them all on this week's menu, intermingled with the tasty grains you've been enjoying for breakfast, the sweet-tasting fruit drinks, fresh vegetables and wonderful fruits you've been enjoying all along.

Anyone for a glass of peach nectar?

Week 4

Life is back to normal already and the month isn't even up yet! Take a good look at this week's menu. It'll give you an idea of the style of eating you'll be following through your lifetime of health. Of course, you won't need the caloric restriction of 1,000, 1,500 or 2,000 calories a day forever. But you'll want to stick with it until you achieve the body weight and look you want.

So what do we have this week? Pancakes, lasagna, potato salad, Art's Brown Apple (yes, that Art is me), Sole Florentine, Fish Creole, just to name a few.

Where's the 20 percent fat? Spread out here and there the way it should be. You'll find a little oil in the Mollen Muffins and in the marinade for the shrimp kabobs. You'll find it in the avocado in the omelet. There's a bit for your toast, muffin or dinner roll. It's in the cheese, in a sandwich.

To stick with a low-fat diet, you've got to remember that it's best to spread the fat throughout each day's menu—not take it straight, like a dollop of butter thrown over a baked potato. By the end of this week, I guarantee that you'll find that a 20-percent-fat diet doesn't seem like a diet at all. It's a good, sensible, natural way of eating.

Take Your Pick

I'm not asking you to give up certain foods. I'm merely asking you to *make wiser choices*, to become more educated about what's good and what isn't good for you. Be creative, try new foods, develop a taste for the Mollen way of life.

So pick a calorie range (the box on page 119 will help you do this) and follow the diet. If three meals a day don't suit you, then save something from breakfast or lunch and eat it for between-meal snacks. If you're still hungry after the meal, then eat an extra piece of fruit or helping of vegetables. These are low enough in fat that it won't make that much of a difference. But an extra helping of fish or chicken will! So if you must have more, think lean—choose fruit or vegetables.

And don't worry if you stumble upon something on the menus that your taste buds just can't handle. If you *can't stand brussels sprouts!* and you're supposed to eat them on Thursday for dinner, just don't eat them. Make a substitution from another day's menu or from the Mollen Method Menu Plan. The calorie plan is listed and so is the serving size. You can easily figure it out.

FOOD GUIDELINES AT A GLANCE

- Eggs are limited to one the first week and two a week thereafter.
- Include a high-fiber food at every meal. Shredded Wheat and Grape-Nuts are great low-fat, high-fiber breakfast choices.
- Eat only whole wheat or other whole grain breads.
- Broth and clear, defatted vegetable soups are good appetite suppressants and can be eaten freely.
- Fresh raw vegetables may be eaten without limitation.
- Low-fat fish, such as fresh halibut, sole, snapper or trout, or canned tuna packed in water can be eaten every day. The serving size should be limited to three to four ounces.
- Shellfish, such as shrimp, crab, lobster, clams and oysters, should be limited to once a week.
- White-meat chicken and turkey without the skin is permitted starting in Week 2.
- Eat only low-fat *plain* yogurt, not the flavored varieties.

- *Only* low-fat cheeses are permitted.
- Whole milk dairy products are not allowed. Low-fat dairy products should be eaten sparingly.
- Eliminate all cream, ice cream and butter. Margarine is permitted in small servings beginning in Week 2. (Butter is high in cholesterol so margarine is a better choice.)
- Fruits can be eaten at every meal. Apples, oranges and cantaloupe are the best choices.
- Fruit preserves and dried fruits, especially raisins, are permitted but should be eaten in moderation because they are high in calories.
- Peanut butter is permitted in moderation—a two-teaspoon serving—starting in Week 3.
- Baked potatoes are allowed but not with butter or sour cream. Use plain, low-fat yogurt, low-fat cottage cheese or Mollenized Sour Cream in place of butter and real sour cream.

The same goes for other foods. If you really hate salmon or can't find red snapper in the market, then substitute another fish. Just remember, substitute fish for fish (I don't mean shellfish), poultry for poultry (and I don't mean game), vegetable for vegetable, fruit for fruit. You've got to be honest if you want the diet to work.

I've used calorie counts and portion control for one reason only. To give you an idea of the calories food contains and to give you a feel for portioning your food.

I despise calorie counting and you probably do, too. But for one month you've got to stick with it; think of it sort of as a crash course in dieting. By the end of the month you'll *know* what a "reasonable portion" should be. When you pick up an apple you'll *know* it's about 80 calories and you'll be able to mentally add it to your day's tally. And as long as you're not gaining weight or gaining fat, you'll be sure you're doing everything right.

Now for a few more features of the diet that I haven't yet mentioned. They have to do with a few things you might think are a big deal in your life (but really aren't). Things like beef, salt, alcohol and caffeine.

The Ban on Beef

I'm sure you've noticed that there isn't a smidgen of beef or its red-meat cousins on any one of the menus or in the Mollen Method Menu Plan. There's a good reason for it. I don't want you to eat any.

Now hold on. Don't go hacking the book with a meat cleaver. I don't want you to give beef up forever. Just for the 30 days of the diet. I do have a good reason for it. Actually many good reasons.

Reason number one is that beef is high in fat and high in calories. And from talks with my patients I've discovered beef is something people don't eat in 2-ounce portions. Does a 12-ounce or even a 16-ounce steak sound incredible? Not to beef lovers. But a 12-ounce sirloin steak weighs in at 1,600 calories, more than some people consume in an entire day. Talk about protein overload. Even if you cut away the visible fat from that steak, you'll still be left with 800 calories—and 47 percent of these calories come from fat.

So I'd like you to give up red meat for the month. Honest, it won't kill you. It probably won't even bother you. I'm always amused by the contrast between my patients' reactions when I tell them they can't have red meat for a month and their comments after the month is over.

"You know, I never missed it" is a common comment. "I just don't care for red meat the way I used to" is another. "It makes me feel so *full*" is yet another.

When you do go back to red meat, take it in small doses. I don't mean cutting back from a 12-ounce to a 3-ounce portion. I mean learn how to make a little go a long way. Braise it in stews with plenty of vegetables. Skewer it on shish kabobs with onions, green peppers and tomatoes, or make it part of a casserole. Find ways to make a whole meal using only a small amount of meat. I'll bet you find you like it better that way.

Hold the Salt

Take a look at the menus in this chapter. They sound good, don't they? Plenty of spices to make them tasty. What you won't find—except in a very few instances where I felt it essential—is salt.

Along with cutting back on beef, I'd also like you to learn to live with eating less salt.

You've no doubt heard by now that too much salt contributes to high blood pressure, a major risk factor for heart disease. And since this is not just a reducing diet, but a *health* diet, I want you to learn to live with less salt.

Studies have shown, and my patients will attest, that cutting back on salt is really quite easy to do. Take away the salt shaker and in a very short while you will no longer feel deprived of salt; in fact, the reverse will happen. Foods will start to taste too salty.

So be your own patrol and start monitoring your salt intake. Never salt the foods you're cooking and never leave a salt shaker on the table. Make it an effort to salt your food, not a convenience. For example, store it in a closet away from the stove. Then, if you really feel you need salt, you'll have to walk across the room to get it. And don't worry about not getting enough salt. You'll get plenty of it naturally in the foods you'll be eating.

Fitting Alcohol into Your Life

Alcohol is an area in which my diet really differs from others. I allow it. But for one week—for just seven days—I'm going to ask you to give it up. If in Week 2 you feel you simply must have your Saturday night cocktail, well go ahead. But limit it to one. In Weeks 3 and 4, you can have two drinks a week. After that your alcohol intake is under your own control. All I ask is this: Keep a sensible attitude about it.

I want you to become acutely aware of the calories in your favorite drinks and realize how quickly they can add up. A 3-ounce glass of wine, for

(Continued on page 152)

MOLLEN METHOD MENU PLAN
Week 1
5% Calories from Fat

Allowed (listed in serving sizes)	Off Limits	Servings per Day (according to diet plan)
MILK (includes milk, yogurt and ice cream)		
Skim milk, 1 cup	1% milk	1,000 calories: 1 serving
Powdered skim milk (nonfat dry milk), before adding liquid, 1/3 cup	2% milk	1,500 calories: 2 servings
Skim buttermilk, 1 cup	Whole milk	2,000 calories: 3 servings
Plain, low-fat yogurt, 1 cup	Whole-milk beverages (includes malts and shakes made with ice cream and milk)	
	Chocolate-flavored milks	
	Yogurt made from whole milk and 2% milk	
	All flavored yogurts	
	Ice cream	
	Ice milk	
FRUITS AND FRUIT JUICES (Fruits may be fresh, dried, frozen, canned, cooked or raw. Juices may be canned, frozen or freshly squeezed.)		
Apples, 1 small	All fruits with sugar added:	1,000 calories: 4 servings
Apricots, 4 halves	Fruits canned in syrup	1,500 calories: 7 servings
Bananas, 1/2 small	Sweetened frozen fruits	2,000 calories: 10 servings
Cantaloupe, 1/4 small	Sweetened fruit juices	
Cherries, 10 large	All fruits high in fat:	
Dates, 2	Avocados	
Figs, 1	Olives	
Grapefruit, 1/2		
Grapes, 12		
Oranges, 1 small		
Peaches, 1 medium		
Pears, 1 small		
Pineapple, cubed, 1/2 cup		

(Continued)

MOLLEN METHOD MENU PLAN – *Continued*
Week 1

Allowed (listed in serving sizes)	Off Limits	Servings per Day (according to diet plan)
FRUITS AND FRUIT JUICES – *Continued*		
Plums (prunes), 2 medium		
Raisins, 2 tablespoons		
Watermelon, cubed, 1 cup		
Apple juice, 1/3 cup		
Grape juice, 1/4 cup		
Orange juice, 1/2 cup		
Prune juice, 1/4 cup		
VEGETABLES AND VEGETABLE JUICES		
Asparagus	All other nonstarchy vegetables	1,000, 1,500 and 2,000 calories: unlimited
Bean sprouts		
Beets		
Broccoli		

Allowed (listed in serving sizes)	Off Limits	Servings per Day (according to diet plan)
VEGETABLES AND VEGETABLE JUICES – *Continued*		
Tomatoes		
Turnips		
Watercress		
Zucchini		
Tomato juice		
Vegetable juices		
STARCHY VEGETABLES		
Corn, 1/3 cup	All fresh or frozen vegetables prepared with additional fat	1,000 calories: 2 servings
Corn on the cob, 1 small	French fries	1,500 calories: 3 servings
Lima beans, 1/2 cup	Potato chips	2,000 calories: 4 servings
Parsnips, 2/3 cup		
Peas, green, canned, fresh or frozen, 1/2 cup		
Potatoes, white, 1 small		

Brussels sprouts
Cabbage
Carrots
Cauliflower
Celery
Chicory
Chinese cabbage
Cucumbers
Eggplant
Endive
Escarole
Greens:
  Beet
  Chard
  Collard
  Dandelion
  Kale
  Mustard
  Spinach
  Turnip
Lettuce
Mushrooms
Okra
Onions
Parsley
Peppers, green
Radishes
Rhubarb
Rutabagas
String beans, green or yellow
Summer squash

Potatoes, mashed, ½ cup
Pumpkin, ¾ cup
Winter squash, acorn or butternut, ½ cup
Yams or sweet potatoes, ¼ cup
Dried beans, peas and lentils, cooked, ½ cup

BREADS AND PASTA

Whole wheat bread, 1 slice
Rye bread, 1 slice
Pumpernickel bread, 1 slice
Whole wheat English muffins, ½
Whole wheat dinner rolls, 1
Whole wheat crackers, 6
Melba toast, 4 slices
Rye wafers, 4
Spaghetti, cooked, ½ cup
Macaroni, cooked, ½ cup

Breads made with eggs, cream, cheese and nuts
Breads containing fat:
  Sweet rolls
  Biscuits
  Muffins
  Popovers
  Corn bread
  Pancakes
  Waffles
  French toast
Crackers high in fat:
  All round butter-type
  Bacon-flavored
  Cheese-flavored
  Onion-flavored

1,000 calories: 3 servings
1,500 calories: 4 servings
2,000 calories: 5 servings

(Continued)

MOLLEN METHOD MENU PLAN–Continued
Week 1

Allowed (listed in serving sizes)	Off Limits	Servings per Day (according to diet plan)
GRAINS		
Cereals made from barley, bulgur, oats and wheat, ½ to 1 cup Cooked cereals, ½ cup Ready-to-eat unsweetened cereals, ¾ cup Rice, ½ cup	All other cereals and grains	1,000 calories: 1 serving 1,500 calories: 2 servings 2,000 calories: 2 servings
MEATS AND FISH		
Fish, any kind, baked, broiled or poached, except shrimp	All meats: Beef Veal Lamb Mutton Pork Chicken	1,000 calories: 2–3 ounces 1,500 calories: 3–4 ounces 2,000 calories: 3–4 ounces
FATS		
None	Butter Margarine Oils Shortening Lard Meat fat Heavy cream Sour cream Cream cheese Cream sauces Gravies Mayonnaise Salad dressings made with fat	None
NUTS AND SEEDS		
None	All nuts and seeds	None

Allowed	Avoid	Amount
	Turkey	
	Frankfurters	
	Sausage	
	Bacon	
	Luncheon meats	
	Organ meats	
	Sweetbreads	
	Gizzards	
	All game	
	All fried and breaded fish	
	Fish canned in oil	
	Shrimp	

EGGS

Allowed	Avoid	Amount
Egg whites, 2	Egg yolks	1,000, 1,500 and 2,000 calories: 1 serving
Liquid egg substitute, ¼ cup		

CHEESES

Allowed	Avoid	Amount
Low-fat cottage cheese, ½ cup	Cheeses made from whole milk or cream	1,000 calories: 1 serving
Part-skim ricotta, ¼ cup		1,500 calories: 1 serving
Uncreamed or low-fat cheeses made partly from skim milk, 1 ounce		2,000 calories: 2 servings
Farmer or pot cheese, 1 ounce		
Part-skim mozzarella, 1 ounce		

SOUPS

Allowed	Avoid	Amount
Bouillon, fat-free broth and clear vegetable soups	All others	1,000, 1,500 and 2,000 calories: unlimited

BEVERAGES

Allowed	Avoid	Amount
Decaffeinated coffee	All caffeine-containing beverages:	1,000, 1,500 and 2,000 calories: unlimited
Herbal tea	Coffee	
Unsweetened carbonated beverages, such as club soda	Tea	
Cereal beverages	Cocoa	
	Soft drinks	
	Sugared drinks	
	Artificially sweetened beverages	

ALCOHOL

Allowed	Avoid	Amount
None	All alcoholic beverages	None

CONDIMENTS

Allowed	Avoid	Amount
Herbs	Salt	1,000, 1,500 and 2,000 calories: unlimited
Spices	Condiments containing sodium	
Vinegar	Artificial sweeteners	

(Continued)

MOLLEN METHOD MENU PLAN – *Continued*
Week 1

Allowed (listed in serving sizes)	Off Limits	Servings per Day (according to diet plan)
DESSERTS		
Apple butter, 1 tablespoon	Custards	1,000 calories: 1 serving
Jam, jelly or marmalade, 1 teaspoon	Puddings	1,500 calories: 2 servings, 4 times a week
Sugar, honey or syrup, 1 teaspoon	Ice cream	2,000 calories: 2 servings
	Canned fruits in syrup	
	Commercial cakes	
	Pies	

Allowed (listed in serving sizes)	Off Limits	Servings per Day (according to diet plan)
DESSERTS – *Continued*		
	Cookies and mixes	
	Candy	
	Chocolate	

Week 2
10% Calories from Fat

Allowed (listed in serving sizes)	Off Limits	Servings per Day (according to diet plan)	Allowed (listed in serving sizes)	Off Limits	Servings per Day (according to diet plan)
MILK (includes milk, yogurt and ice cream)			**FRUITS AND FRUIT JUICES (Fruits may be fresh, dried, frozen, canned, cooked or raw. Juices may be canned, frozen or freshly squeezed.)**		
Skim milk, 1 cup	1% milk	1,000 calories: 1 serving	Apples, 1 small	All fruits with sugar added:	1,000 calories: 4 servings
Powdered skim milk (nonfat dry milk), before adding liquid, ⅓ cup	2% milk	1,500 calories: 2 servings	Apricots, 4 halves	Fruits canned in syrup	1,500 calories: 7 servings
Skim buttermilk, 1 cup	Whole milk	2,000 calories: 3 servings	Bananas, ½ small	Sweetened frozen fruits	2,000 calories: 10 servings
Plain, low-fat yogurt, 1 cup	Whole-milk beverages (includes malts and shakes made with ice cream and milk)		Cantaloupe, ¼ small	Sweetened fruit juices	
	Chocolate-flavored milks		Cherries, 10 large	All fruits high in fat:	
	Yogurt made from whole milk and 2% milk		Dates, 2	Avocados	
	All flavored yogurts		Figs, 1	Olives	
	Ice cream		Grapefruit, ½		
	Ice milk		Grapes, 12		
			Oranges, 1 small		
			Peaches, 1 medium		
			Pears, 1 small		
			Pineapple, cubed, ½ cup		

(Continued)

MOLLEN METHOD MENU PLAN – *Continued*
Week 2

Allowed (listed in serving sizes)	Off Limits	Servings per Day (according to diet plan)
FRUITS AND FRUIT JUICES – *Continued*		
Plums (prunes), 2 medium		
Raisins, 2 tablespoons		
Watermelon, cubed, 1 cup		
Apple juice, $\frac{1}{3}$ cup		
Grape juice, $\frac{1}{4}$ cup		
Orange juice, $\frac{1}{2}$ cup		
Prune juice, $\frac{1}{4}$ cup		
VEGETABLES AND VEGETABLE JUICES		
Asparagus	All other nonstarchy vegetables	1,000, 1,500 and 2,000 calories: unlimited
Bean sprouts		
Beets		
Broccoli		
VEGETABLES AND VEGETABLE JUICES – *Continued*		
Tomatoes		
Turnips		
Watercress		
Zucchini		
Tomato juice		
Vegetable juices		
STARCHY VEGETABLES		
Corn, $\frac{1}{3}$ cup	All fresh or frozen vegetables prepared with additional fat	1,000 calories: 2 servings
Corn on the cob, 1 small	French fries	1,500 calories: 3 servings
Lima beans, $\frac{1}{2}$ cup	Potato chips	2,000 calories: 4 servings
Parsnips, $\frac{2}{3}$ cup		
Peas, green, canned, fresh or frozen, $\frac{1}{2}$ cup		

Brussels sprouts
Cabbage
Carrots
Cauliflower
Celery
Chicory
Chinese cabbage
Cucumbers
Eggplant
Endive
Escarole
Greens:
  Beet
  Chard
  Collard
  Dandelion
  Kale
  Mustard
  Spinach
  Turnip
Lettuce
Mushrooms
Okra
Onions
Parsley
Peppers, green
Radishes
Rhubarb
Rutabagas
String beans, green or yellow
Summer squash

Potatoes, white, 1 small
Potatoes, mashed, ½ cup
Pumpkin, ¾ cup
Winter squash, acorn or butternut, ½ cup
Yams or sweet potatoes, ¼ cup
Dried beans, peas and lentils, cooked, ½ cup

BREADS AND PASTA

Whole wheat bread, 1 slice
Rye bread, 1 slice
Pumpernickel bread, 1 slice
Whole wheat English muffins, ½
Whole wheat dinner rolls, 1
Whole wheat crackers, 6
Melba toast, 4 slices
Rye wafers, 4
Spaghetti, cooked, ½ cup
Macaroni, cooked, ½ cup

Breads made with eggs, cream, cheese and nuts
Crackers high in fat:
All round butter-type
Bacon-flavored
Cheese-flavored
Onion-flavored

1,000 calories: 3 servings
1,500 calories: 4 servings
2,000 calories: 5 servings

(Continued)

MOLLEN METHOD MENU PLAN—*Continued*
Week 2

Allowed (listed in serving sizes)	Off Limits	Servings per Day (according to diet plan)
BREADS AND PASTA—*Continued*		
The following contain fat and are limited to 2–3 servings per week: Biscuits, 1, 2-inch diameter; Muffins, 1; Corn bread, 1 slice; Pancakes, 1, 5 inches by ½ inch; Waffles, 1, 5 inches by ½ inch; French toast, 1 slice		
GRAINS		
Cereals made from barley, bulgur, oats and wheat, ½ to 1 cup	All other cereals and grains	1,000 calories: 1 serving; 1,500 calories: 2 servings
EGGS		
Egg whites, 2; Liquid egg substitute, ¼ cup; Whole eggs, 1-2 per week	None	1,000, 1,500 and 2,000 calories: 1 serving
CHEESES		
Low-fat cottage cheese, ½ cup; Part-skim ricotta, ¼ cup; Uncreamed or low-fat cheeses made partly from skim milk, 1 ounce; Farmer or pot cheese, 1 ounce; Part-skim mozzarella, 1 ounce	Cheeses made from whole milk or cream	1,000 calories: 1 serving; 1,500 calories: 1 serving; 2,000 calories: 2 servings

FATS

Margarine, 1 teaspoon	Butter	1,000, 1,500 and 2,000 calories: 1 serving
Oils, 1 teaspoon	Shortening	
Low-fat (light) mayonnaise, 1 tablespoon	Lard	
	Meat fat	
	Heavy cream	
	Sour cream	
	Cream cheese	
	Cream sauces	
	Gravies	
	Real mayonnaise	
	Salad dressings made with fat	

NUTS AND SEEDS

None	All nuts and seeds	None

SOUPS

Bouillon, fat-free broth and clear vegetable soups	All others	1,000, 1,500 and 2,000 calories: unlimited

Cooked cereals, ½ cup		2,000 calories: 2 servings
Ready-to-eat unsweetened cereals, ¾ cup		
Rice, ½ cup		

MEATS AND FISH

Fish, any kind, baked, broiled or poached	All red meats:	1,000 calories: 2-3 ounces
The following contain a moderate amount of fat and are limited to 2-3 servings per week:	Beef	1,500 calories: 3-4 ounces
	Veal	2,000 calories: 3-4 ounces
Shrimp, baked, broiled or boiled	Lamb	
Chicken and turkey *without skin*, baked, broiled or poached	Mutton	
	Pork	
	Frankfurters	
	Sausage	
	Bacon	
	Luncheon meats	
	Organ meats	
	Sweetbreads	
	Gizzards	
	Most game	
	All fried and breaded fish and poultry	
	Fish canned in oil	
	Skin of poultry	

(Continued)

MOLLEN METHOD MENU PLAN–Continued
Week 2

Allowed (listed in serving sizes)	Off Limits	Servings per Day (according to diet plan)
BEVERAGES		
Decaffeinated coffee Herbal tea Unsweetened carbonated beverages, such as club soda Cereal beverages	All caffeine-containing beverages: Coffee Tea Cocoa Soft drinks Sugared drinks Artificially sweetened beverages	1,000, 1,500 and 2,000 calories: unlimited
ALCOHOL		
Light beer, 12 ounces Table wine, 3½ ounces	Beer Liqueurs Dessert wines	Limit to 1 drink per week within caloric restrictions

Allowed (listed in serving sizes)	Off Limits	Servings per Day (according to diet plan)
CONDIMENTS		
Herbs Spices Vinegar	Salt Condiments containing sodium Artificial sweeteners	1,000, 1,500 and 2,000 calories: unlimited
DESSERTS		
Apple butter, 1 tablespoon Jam, jelly or marmalade, 1 teaspoon Sugar, honey or syrup, 1 teaspoon	Custards Puddings Ice cream Canned fruits in syrup Commercial cakes Pies Cookies and mixes Candy Chocolate	1,000 calories: 1 serving 1,500 calories: 2 servings, 4 times a week 2,000 calories: 2 servings

(Continued)

Brandy, 1 ounce
Gin, rum or vodka,
1 ounce
Whiskey, 1 ounce
Mixers:
Club soda
Vegetable juices
Unsweetened
fruit juices

Mixers:
Cream
Ice cream
Soft drinks
Sweetened
beverages
Tonic water

MOLLEN METHOD MENU PLAN
Week 3
15% Calories from Fat

Allowed (listed in serving sizes)	Off Limits	Servings per Day (according to diet plan)
MILK (includes milk, yogurt and ice cream)		
Skim milk, 1 cup	1% milk	1,000 calories: 1 serving
Powdered skim milk (nonfat dry milk), before adding liquid, 1/3 cup	2% milk	1,500 calories: 2 servings
Skim buttermilk, 1 cup	Whole milk	2,000 calories: 3 servings
Plain, low-fat yogurt, 1 cup	Whole-milk beverages (includes malts and shakes made with ice cream and milk)	
	Chocolate-flavored milks	
	Yogurt made from whole milk and 2% milk	
	All flavored yogurts	
	Ice cream	
	Ice milk	

Allowed (listed in serving sizes)	Off Limits	Servings per Day (according to diet plan)
FRUITS AND FRUIT JUICES – Continued		
The following are high in fat and are limited to 1-2 servings per week: Avocados, 1/8 Olives, 4		
VEGETABLES AND VEGETABLE JUICES		
Asparagus	All other nonstarchy vegetables	1,000, 1,500 and 2,000 calories: unlimited
Bean sprouts		
Beets		
Broccoli		
Brussels sprouts		
Cabbage		

(Continued)

FRUITS AND FRUIT JUICES (Fruits may be fresh, dried, frozen, canned, cooked or raw. Juices may be canned, frozen or freshly squeezed.)

Apples, 1 small
Apricots, 4 halves
Bananas, ½ small
Cantaloupe, ¼ small
Cherries, 10 large
Dates, 2
Figs, 1
Grapefruit, ½
Grapes, 12
Oranges, 1 small
Peaches, 1 medium
Pears, 1 small
Pineapple, cubed, ½ cup
Plums (prunes), 2 medium
Raisins, 2 tablespoons
Watermelon, cubed, 1 cup
Apple juice, ⅓ cup
Grape juice, ¼ cup
Orange juice, ½ cup
Prune juice, ¼ cup

All fruits with sugar added:
　Fruits canned in syrup
　Sweetened frozen fruits
　Sweetened fruit juices

1,000 calories: 4 servings
1,500 calories: 7 servings
2,000 calories: 10 servings

Carrots
Cauliflower
Celery
Chicory
Chinese cabbage
Cucumbers
Eggplant
Endive
Escarole
Greens:
　Beet
　Chard
　Collard
　Dandelion
　Kale
　Mustard
　Spinach
　Turnip
Lettuce
Mushrooms
Okra
Onions
Parsley
Peppers, green
Radishes
Rhubarb
Rutabagas

MOLLEN METHOD MENU PLAN—Continued
Week 3

Allowed (listed in serving sizes)	Off Limits	Servings per Day (according to diet plan)
VEGETABLES AND VEGETABLE JUICES—Continued		
String beans, green or yellow		
Summer squash		
Tomatoes		
Turnips		
Watercress		
Zucchini		
Tomato juice		
Vegetable juices		
STARCHY VEGETABLES		
Corn, 1/3 cup	All fresh or frozen vegetables prepared with additional fat	1,000 calories: 2 servings
Corn on the cob, 1 small		1,500 calories: 3 servings
Lima beans, 1/2 cup		

Allowed (listed in serving sizes)	Off Limits	Servings per Day (according to diet plan)
BREADS AND PASTA—Continued		
Rye wafers, 4		
Spaghetti, cooked, 1/2 cup		
Macaroni, cooked, 1/2 cup		
The following contain fat and are limited to 2-3 servings per week:		
Biscuits, 1, 2-inch diameter		
Muffins, 1		
Corn bread, 1 slice		
Pancakes, 1, 5 inches by 1/2 inch		

Parsnips, ⅔ cup
Peas, green, canned, fresh or frozen, ½ cup
Potatoes, white, 1 small
Potatoes, mashed, ½ cup
Pumpkin, ¾ cup
Winter squash, acorn or butternut, ½ cup
Yams or sweet potatoes, ¼ cup
Dried beans, peas and lentils, cooked, ½ cup

French fries
Potato chips

2,000 calories: 4 servings

Waffles, 1, 5 inches by ½ inch
French toast, 1 slice

GRAINS

Cereals made from barley, bulgur, oats and wheat, ½ to 1 cup
Cooked cereals, ½ cup
Ready-to-eat unsweetened cereals, ¾ cup
Rice, ½ cup

All other cereals and grains

1,000 calories: 1 serving
1,500 calories: 2 servings
2,000 calories: 2 servings

BREADS AND PASTA

Whole wheat bread, 1 slice
Rye bread, 1 slice
Pumpernickel bread, 1 slice
Whole wheat English muffins, ½
Whole wheat dinner rolls, 1
Whole wheat crackers, 6
Melba toast, 4 slices

Breads made with eggs, cream, cheese and nuts
Crackers high in fat:
All round butter-type
Bacon-flavored
Cheese-flavored
Onion-flavored

1,000 calories: 3 servings
1,500 calories: 4 servings
2,000 calories: 5 servings

MEATS AND FISH

Fish, any kind, baked, broiled or poached
The following contain a moderate amount of fat and are limited to 2-3 servings per week:
Shrimp, baked, broiled or boiled

All red meats:
Beef
Veal
Lamb
Mutton
Pork
Frankfurters
Sausage
Bacon

1,000 calories: 2-3 ounces
1,500 calories: 3-4 ounces
2,000 calories: 3-4 ounces

(Continued)

MOLLEN METHOD MENU PLAN–Continued
Week 3

Allowed (listed in serving sizes)	Off Limits	Servings per Day (according to diet plan)
MEATS AND FISH – Continued		
Chicken and turkey *without skin*, baked, broiled or poached	Luncheon meats Organ meats Sweetbreads Gizzards Most game All fried and breaded fish and poultry Fish canned in oil Skin of poultry	
EGGS		
Egg whites, 2 Liquid egg substitute, ¼ cup Whole eggs, 2–3 per week	None	1,000, 1,500 and 2,000 calories: 1 serving
NUTS AND SEEDS		
Sunflower seeds, 1 tablespoon Almonds, 10 whole Pecans, 2 large Spanish peanuts, 20 Virginia peanuts, 10 Walnuts, 6 small Peanut butter, 1 tablespoon	All other nuts and seeds	1,000, 1,500 and 2,000 calories: limit to 3 servings per week
SOUPS		
Bouillon, fat-free broth and clear vegetable soups	All others	1,000, 1,500 and 2,000 calories: unlimited

CHEESES

Low-fat cottage cheese, ½ cup	Cheeses made from whole milk or cream
Part-skim ricotta, ¼ cup	
Uncreamed or low-fat cheeses made partly from skim milk, 1 ounce	
Farmer or pot cheese, 1 ounce	
Part-skim mozzarella, 1 ounce	

1,000 calories: 1 serving
1,500 calories: 1 serving
2,000 calories: 2 servings

BEVERAGES

Decaffeinated coffee	All caffeine-containing beverages:
Herbal tea	Coffee
Unsweetened carbonated beverages, such as club soda	Tea
Cereal beverages	Cocoa
	Soft drinks
	Sugared drinks
	Artificially sweetened beverages

1,000, 1,500 and 2,000 calories: unlimited

FATS

Margarine, 1 teaspoon	Butter
Oils, 1 teaspoon	Shortening
Italian or French dressing, 1 tablespoon	Lard
Low-fat (light) mayonnaise, 1 tablespoon	Meat fat
Light cream, 2 tablespoons	Heavy cream
	Sour cream
	Cream cheese
	Cream sauces
	Gravies
	Real mayonnaise

1,000 calories: 1 serving
1,500 calories: 1 serving
2,000 calories: 2 servings

ALCOHOL

Light beer, 12 ounces	Beer
Table wine, 3½ ounces	Liqueurs
Brandy, 1 ounce	Dessert wines
Gin, rum or vodka, 1 ounce	Mixers:
Whiskey, 1 ounce	Cream
Mixers:	Ice cream
Club soda	Soft drinks
Vegetable juices	Sweetened beverages
Unsweetened fruit juices	Tonic water

Limit to 1-2 drinks per week within caloric restrictions

(Continued)

MOLLEN METHOD MENU PLAN–Continued
Week 3

Allowed (listed in serving sizes)	Off Limits	Servings per Day (according to diet plan)
CONDIMENTS		
Herbs Spices Vinegar	Salt Condiments containing sodium Artificial sweeteners	1,000, 1,500 and 2,000 calories: unlimited
DESSERTS		
Apple butter, 1 tablespoon Jam, jelly or marmalade, 1 teaspoon Sugar, honey or syrup, 1 teaspoon	Custards Puddings Ice cream Canned fruits in syrup Commercial cakes Pies Cookies and mixes Candy Chocolate	1,000 calories: 1 serving 1,500 calories: 2 servings, 4 times a week 2,000 calories: 2 servings

Week 4
20% Calories from Fat

Allowed (listed in serving sizes)	Off Limits	Servings per Day (according to diet plan)
MILK (includes milk, yogurt and ice cream)		
Skim milk, 1 cup	1% milk	1,000 calories: 1 serving
Powdered skim milk (nonfat dry milk), before adding liquid, 1/3 cup	2% milk	1,500 calories: 2 servings
Skim buttermilk, 1 cup	Whole milk	2,000 calories: 3 servings
Plain, low-fat yogurt, 1 cup	Whole-milk beverages (includes malts and shakes made with ice cream and milk)	*Maintenance diet: unlimited*
	Chocolate-flavored milks	
	Yogurt made from whole milk and 2% milk	
	All flavored yogurts	
	Ice cream	
	Ice milk	
FRUITS AND FRUIT JUICES (Fruits may be fresh, dried, frozen, canned, cooked or raw. Juices may be canned, frozen or freshly squeezed.)		
Apples, 1 small	All fruits with sugar added:	1,000 calories: 4 servings
Apricots, 4 halves	Fruits canned in syrup	1,500 calories: 7 servings
Bananas, 1/2 small	Sweetened frozen fruits	2,000 calories: 10 servings
Cantaloupe, 1/4 small	Sweetened fruit juices	*Maintenance diet: unlimited*
Cherries, 10 large		
Dates, 2		
Figs, 1		
Grapefruit, 1/2		
Grapes, 12		
Oranges, 1 small		
Peaches, 1 medium		
Pears, 1 small		
Pineapple, cubed, 1/2 cup		
Plums (prunes), 2 medium		

(Continued)

MOLLEN METHOD MENU PLAN – *Continued*
Week 4

Allowed (listed in serving sizes)	Off Limits	Servings per Day (according to diet plan)
FRUITS AND FRUIT JUICES — *Continued*		
Raisins, 2 table-spoons		
Watermelon, cubed, 1 cup		
Apple juice, 1/3 cup		
Grape juice, 1/4 cup		
Orange juice, 1/2 cup		
Prune juice, 1/4 cup		
The following are high in fat and are limited to 1-2 servings per week:		
Avocados, 1/8		
Olives, 4		
VEGETABLES AND VEGETABLE JUICES — *Continued*		
Peppers, green		
Radishes		
Rhubarb		
Rutabagas		
String beans, green or yellow		
Summer squash		
Tomatoes		
Turnips		
Watercress		
Zucchini		
Tomato juice		
Vegetable juices		

VEGETABLES AND VEGETABLE JUICES		STARCHY VEGETABLES	
Asparagus	All other nonstarchy vegetables	Corn, ⅓ cup	All fresh or frozen vegetables pre- pared with additional fat
Bean sprouts	1,000, 1,500 and 2,000 calories: unlimited	Corn on the cob, 1 small	French fries
Beets		Lima beans, ½ cup	Potato chips
Broccoli		Parsnips, ⅔ cup	
Brussels sprouts		Peas, green, canned, fresh or frozen, ½ cup	1,000 calories: 2 servings
Cabbage			1,500 calories: 3 servings
Carrots		Potatoes, white, 1 small	2,000 calories: 4 servings
Cauliflower		Potatoes, mashed, ½ cup	*Maintenance diet:* *unlimited*
Celery		Pumpkin, ¾ cup	
Chicory		Winter squash, acorn or butternut, ½ cup	
Chinese cabbage		Yams or sweet potatoes, ¼ cup	
Cucumbers		Dried beans, peas and lentils, cooked, ½ cup	
Eggplant			
Endive			
Escarole			
Greens:			
Beet			
Chard			
Collard			
Dandelion			
Kale			
Mustard			
Spinach			
Turnip			
Lettuce			
Mushrooms			
Okra			
Onions			
Parsley			

(Continued)

MOLLEN METHOD MENU PLAN–*Continued*
Week 4

Allowed (listed in serving sizes)	Off Limits	Servings per Day (according to diet plan)
BREADS AND PASTA		
Whole wheat bread, 1 slice Rye bread, 1 slice Pumpernickel bread, 1 slice Whole wheat English muffins, ½ Whole wheat dinner rolls, 1 Whole wheat crackers, 6 Melba toast, 4 slices Rye wafers, 4 Spaghetti, cooked, ½ cup Macaroni, cooked, ½ cup	Breads made with eggs, cream, cheese and nuts Crackers high in fat: All round butter-type Bacon-flavored Cheese-flavored Onion-flavored	1,000 calories: 3 servings 1,500 calories: 4 servings 2,000 calories: 5 servings *Maintenance diet: unlimited*
MEATS AND FISH		
Fish, any kind, baked, broiled or poached *The following contain a moderate amount of fat and are limited to 2-3 servings per week:* Shrimp, baked, broiled or boiled Chicken and turkey *without skin,* baked, broiled or poached	All red meats: Beef Veal Lamb Mutton Pork Frankfurters Sausage Bacon Luncheon meats Organ meats Sweetbreads Gizzards Most game All fried and breaded fish and poultry Fish canned in oil Skin of poultry	1,000 calories: 2-3 ounces 1,500 calories: 3-4 ounces 2,000 calories: 3-4 ounces *Maintenance diet: limit to 4 ounces per day*

The following contain fat and are limited to 2-3 servings per week:

Biscuits, 1, 2-inch diameter
Muffins, 1
Corn bread, 1 slice
Pancakes, 1, 5 inches by ½ inch
Waffles, 1, 5 inches by ½ inch
French toast, 1 slice

GRAINS

Cereals made from barley, bulgur, oats and wheat, ½ to 1 cup Cooked cereals, ½ cup Ready-to-eat unsweetened cereals, ¾ cup Rice, ½ cup	All other cereals and grains	1,000 calories: 1 serving 1,500 calories: 2 servings 2,000 calories: 2 servings *Maintenance diet: unlimited*

EGGS

Egg whites, 2 Liquid egg substitute, ¼ cup Whole eggs, 2-3 per week	None	1,000, 1,500 and 2,000 calories: 1 serving *Maintenance diet: unlimited* *Whole eggs: limit to 2-3 times a week*

CHEESES

Low-fat cottage cheese, ½ cup Part-skim ricotta, ¼ cup Uncreamed or low-fat cheeses made partly from skim milk, 1 ounce Farmer or pot cheese, 1 ounce Part-skim mozzarella, 1 ounce	Cheeses made from whole milk or cream	1,000 calories: 1 serving 1,500 calories: 1 serving 2,000 calories: 2 servings *Maintenance diet: limit to 2 servings*

(Continued)

MOLLEN METHOD MENU PLAN—Continued
Week 4

Allowed (listed in serving sizes)	Off Limits	Servings per Day (according to diet plan)
FATS		
Margarine, 1 teaspoon	Butter	1,000 calories: 2 servings
Oils, 1 teaspoon	Shortening	1,500 calories: 2 servings
Italian or French dressing, 1 tablespoon	Lard	2,000 calories: 3 servings
Low-fat (light) mayonnaise, 1 tablespoon	Meat fat	*Maintenance diet: 3 servings*
Light cream, 2 tablespoons	Heavy cream	
	Sour cream	
	Cream cheese	
	Cream sauces	
	Gravies	
	Real mayonnaise	
NUTS AND SEEDS		
Sunflower seeds, 1 tablespoon	All other nuts and seeds	1,000, 1,500 and 2,000 calories: limit to 3 servings per week
Almonds, 10 whole		
Pecans, 2 large		
Spanish peanuts, 20		

Allowed (listed in serving sizes)	Off Limits	Servings per Day (according to diet plan)
ALCOHOL		
Light beer, 12 ounces	Beer	Limit to 1-2 drinks per week within caloric restrictions
Table wine, 3½ ounces	Liqueurs	
Brandy, 1 ounce	Dessert wines	
Gin, rum or vodka, 1 ounce	Mixers:	
Whiskey, 1 ounce	Cream	
Mixers:	Ice cream	
Club soda	Soft drinks	
Unsweetened fruit juices	Sweetened beverages	
Vegetable juices	Tonic water	
CONDIMENTS		
Herbs	Salt	1,000, 1,500 and 2,000 calories: unlimited
Spices	Condiments containing sodium	
Vinegar	Artificial sweeteners	

Virginia peanuts, 10		
Walnuts, 6 small		
Peanut butter, 1 tablespoon		*Maintenance diet: 3 servings per week*

SOUPS

Bouillon, fat-free broth and clear vegetable soups	All others	1,000, 1,500 and 2,000 calories: unlimited

BEVERAGES

Decaffeinated coffee	All caffeine-containing beverages:	1,000, 1,500 and 2,000 calories: unlimited
Herbal tea	Coffee	
Unsweetened carbonated beverages, such as club soda	Tea	
Cereal beverages	Cocoa	
	Soft drinks	
	Sugared drinks	
	Artificially sweetened beverages	

DESSERTS

Apple butter, 1 tablespoon	Custards	1,000 calories: 1 serving
Jam, jelly or marmalade, 1 teaspoon	Puddings	1,500 calories: 2 servings, 4 times a week
Sugar, honey or syrup, 1 teaspoon	Ice cream	2,000 calories: 2 servings
	Canned fruits in syrup	*Maintenance diet: 2 servings per day*
	Commercial cakes	
	Pies	
	Cookies and mixes	
	Candy	
	Chocolate	

THE MOLLEN MANHATTAN

One of the most annoying things to a weight watcher (or to anyone for that matter) is to go to a party and have people constantly try to put a cocktail in your hand when you don't really want one. I've found that the best way to avoid this problem is to already have a cocktail in hand—one that's low in calories and contains no alcohol. I call it the Mollen Manhattan and it's only 24 calories a drink. Here's the recipe:

Mollen Manhattan

4 ounces club soda
1 teaspoon bitters
1 maraschino cherry

Combine the club soda and bitters in a small martini pitcher and gently stir. Pour into a low ball glass filled to the brim with chopped ice. Add the cherry and drink.
Cheers!

---

instance, has 75 calories. Light beer runs about 90 to 110 calories for a 12-ounce bottle and regular beer contains 140 to 180 calories. Mixed drinks can run anywhere from 125 calories for a generous whiskey and water to 342 calories for a glass of eggnog. It's true alcohol doesn't contain fat, but it doesn't contain much of anything else either. Almost no vitamins or minerals. Just empty calories. So keep your alcohol consumption under control.

The second most important thing to remember is to pace yourself. As calorie count goes up with consumption, willpower goes down. Alcohol tends to make you eat more, putting you at risk for weight gain. Also, that logy feeling you get the day after drinking is not conducive to exercise. My suggestion for optimum health after you've reached your weight-loss goal is to limit your drinks to no more than two a day. As for myself? I drink light beer only and have no more than one or two a week.

Caffeine—The Word Is Caution

Caffeine is hard to avoid. It seems to be everywhere—in colas, coffee, chocolate, even medicine. But coffee, by far, is the most abundantly consumed caffeine-containing product.

When patients come to me for a diet I expect them to give up caffeine. Why? Because too many people use it as a crutch. They use it to wake up in the morning, to get their work done in the afternoon and to keep them from eating. They drink maybe two or three cups of coffee at home in the morning, and another two or three after they arrive at work. Then after lunch they head over to the pop machine and drink two colas in the afternoon. After dinner it's more coffee. And they're forever complaining about "having insomnia again last night." No wonder! It's all the caffeine.

Too much caffeine can cause nervousness, anxiety, irritability, insomnia, abnormal heartbeats and heart palpitations. It even makes it more difficult for you to follow a diet because it has a direct effect on your central nervous system. Sure it will suppress your appetite for a while, just like an amphetamine. But when it wears off—look out—you'll really have an appetite! And you may find your appetite hard to control.

So try to eliminate caffeine for a while. Once you've embarked on this new way of living, go for a clean break. Instead of coffee, drink decaffeinated coffee or herbal teas. And give up the diet pop. I'm sure you'll find club soda or seltzer water a lot more refreshing.

Milk and Other Dairy Products

Milk is good for you, yet bad for you, too. We need it for strong bones—just a glass a day provides us with an abundance of calcium. The same goes for its cousins, cheese and yogurt. With all the vitamins and minerals these foods contain, we'd be foolhardy not to include them in our daily diet. But, as I said, they do have their bad side: Dairy products have plenty of fat!

A total of 48 percent of the calories in a glass of whole milk comes from fat; 47 percent of the calories in a cup of whole-milk yogurt comes from fat; and one ounce of most whole-milk cheeses hovers in the 60 to 80 percent bracket. That's way too high if you want to keep your fat intake to 20 percent.

But the food industry has done us a favor by defatting dairy products. So milk, cheese and yogurt can fit quite nicely into your diet plan.

The buy word for dairy products is low fat. Milk should *always* be skim. At 88 calories a cup, only 4.5 percent comes from fat. One percent milk is 102 calories a cup with 22 percent of the calories coming from fat, and 2 percent milk is 121 calories a cup with 34 percent from fat. As you can see, skim milk is a much better deal.

Yogurt? Buy it plain and low fat. Here you're only dealing with 127 calories a cup and 21 percent calories from fat.

The same goes for cheese. You'll find more and more cheeses on the market these days with a low-fat or part-skim label. Eat these only. My patients have found them really quite tasty. How much fat can you save? Almost half the amount you'd get in whole-milk cheese.

TIPS FOR DINING OUT

There's no need to say "Sorry, I'm on a diet" when someone asks you to dinner. Dining out can be an eating pleasure not a diet destroyer —as long as you approach it with the right attitude. Telling yourself "I'm going to get my money's worth," for instance, is the *wrong* attitude. But saying "I can have a nice, leisurely meal and enjoy myself *more* by eating light" is the right attitude. Here are some tips to help you go about it:

- Speak up. *Always* ask the waiter or waitress how a dish is prepared. What sounds like lean cuisine may turn out to be mean cuisine when it shows up on your plate swimming in butter or cream.
- Never put yourself in the position of feeling obliged to "eat the whole thing." If a serving size is large (and in a restaurant servings usually are), divide the portion in half and push the rest aside (or take it home for another meal). If you think you're going to be tempted to clean your plate, then ask the waiter to wrap up half *before* you start to eat. You might get an odd glance but, remember, they're *your* calories.
- Measure your foods at home until you get a sense of portion size by just looking at a dish. This will help to keep you from deceiving yourself when you're mentally counting calories.
- Have an idea of what you're going to eat before you enter the restaurant (fish is always a good choice), and read only that section of the menu. Menus were designed to whet your appetite. Why go through all that torture?
- Always ask that dressings and sauces be served on the side. This way you—not the chef—get to control your calorie intake.
- When the waiter brings the bread ask him to take the butter away.
- When it's time for dessert order fresh fruit. You probably won't find it on the menu but most restaurants have it on hand.
- Never skip breakfast or lunch because you're going out for dinner that evening. It'll only work against you. You'll end up famished and eat more.
- Drinking alcohol prior to eating will increase your appetite so limit pre-meal cocktails to one.
- If you eat at the same restaurant frequently, have the maître d' keep your favorite low-calorie salad dressing or Mollenized Sour Cream for your baked potatoes in the kitchen's refrigerator.

- A light snack of raw vegetables or an apple before dinner will help curb your appetite and put you more in control. Long delays in meal service can do a job on your willpower.
- Order a la carte instead of full dinners. This way you only get what you ask for.
- When dining with a close friend, order appetizers and salad and split the main course.

Should your meal not go as planned, remember the diet is not over. You are learning new habits, which have to be practiced. As Scarlett O'Hara said, Tomorrow is another day . . . .

Here are some other do's and don'ts worth remembering:

Appetizers

Do: Order vegetable juices, unsweetened fruit juices, uncreamed soups, consommés, crudités and so on. Lemon juice may be used as a flavoring. Fresh shellfish, such as shrimp, crab or lobster, served cold with a bit of cocktail sauce, vinaigrette or just sprinkled with lemon are fine once in a while as long as you keep the rest of the meal light. Better yet, order an appetizer as your main course.

Don't: Order creamed soups, bisques, pâtés, soufflés, mousses or pasta to start a meal. It's just too much too soon.

Main Courses

Do: Stick with either fish or poultry roasted, baked, broiled, grilled or poached. Trim off any fat. Request that any sauce be served on the side. Use it for *light* dipping instead of pouring it on top.

Don't: Order anything fried, sautéed, stewed, braised, creamed, breaded or served with gravy. Forget beef. Restaurant portions are just too large. Restaurant cuts also usually contain a higher percentage of fat.

Sandwiches

Do: Order sandwiches of fish (but not fried), turkey breast or chicken. Ask for whole wheat bread, not white bread. Request toppings of lettuce, tomatoes, onions, radishes or other fresh vegetables. Use mustard instead of mayonnaise or other sandwich dressings.

Don't: Order hot gravy-covered sandwiches, club sandwiches, sandwiches filled with cream cheese, sandwiches grilled in fat or fried, or chicken or tuna "salad" sandwiches. The "salad" means mayonnaise, which means 98 percent fat.

(Continued)

TIPS FOR DINING OUT–*Continued*

Potatoes

Do: Order baked, mashed, boiled or steamed potatoes. Use plain, low-fat yogurt or low-fat cottage cheese in place of sour cream as a topping. Or order some mixed vegetables, put them on top of the potato and make that your main course.

Don't: Order home fries, french fries or creamed or scalloped potatoes.

Vegetables

Do: Order stewed, steamed, boiled or baked vegetables. Ask that butter not be added.

Don't: Order creamed, scalloped, au gratin, fried or sautéed vegetables. Stay away from casseroles.

Salad and Salad Dressings

Do: Order only green salad (dark greens are preferable) without dress-ings. Or order fresh fruit salad. Use vinegar or lemon juice as seasoning.

Don't: Order coleslaw, potato salad, molded gelatin salad or salads that contain nuts or cheese.

Breads

Do: Request dark bread instead of white and eat it plain.

Don't: Eat sweet rolls, sweet breads, nut breads, coffee cake, fried breads. If the waiter puts them on the table, ask him to take them away.

Beverages

Do: Order skim milk, unsweetened fruit juices, vegetable juices, club soda, iced herb tea or decaffeinated beverages.

Don't: Order chocolate milk, cocoa and milk drinks, such as shakes or malts, or regular soft drinks.

Fight Fat with Fiber

The grains, cereals, fruits and vegetables you'll be eating every day on the Mollen Method have one thing in common–fiber. Fiber is an extraordi-nary fat fighter. Because it is usually unrefined, fiber can be filling yet still reasonably low in calories.

Fiber-rich foods also offer quality calories–you get a high premium in vitamins and minerals for the small amount of calories these foods contain.

Another benefit of fiber is the ease with which it travels through your digestive tract. Fiber has the ability to pick up moisture as it moves through your intestines, taking calories and fat with it as it passes out of your system. It gives fat little opportunity to snuggle up to fat cells. The fat simply gets carried away.

A special kind of fiber–bran–is particularly beneficial to this bulking action. That's why I emphasize whole grain breads and whole grain cereals on this diet. They provide the bulk you need to keep calorie-laden foods on the move. For the same reason, I've included at least one apple a day on your menu plans. Whole grains and apples. Together they'll keep your digestive tract on the right track.

I Bet My Patients Pounds

I am so convinced that this diet works that for years now I've been betting money on it. I tell my patients that as long as they're losing pounds they don't have to pay for their visits each time they come to my office for their diet consultation and weigh in. It's worked like a charm.

In one year alone, my patients lost a total of 2,000 pounds and I lost $20,000 in patient revenue. A patient who loses 100 pounds gains $1,000 in free doctor visits. I have more than one patient who's done just that.

But I don't mind the loss of income at all. What I've lost in money I've more than made up in a lifetime of gratitude from the hundreds of thin and healthy people who walk out of my office for the last time.

I'd love to make the same bet with you. Unfortunately, that's impossible. But I've found it such a wonderful motivation tool, I feel it might be worthwhile for you to try it on your own.

Make a bet with your spouse, a friend or your boss, or get a group of friends and go on the Mollen Method together. If you don't want to bet money, make it a weekend getaway, a nice vacation trip, a night on the town, or a new wardrobe (which you'll need when you drop your excess weight). Small incentives can reap big rewards. Listen to what a few of my patients had to say about this:

"My husband was thrilled with me when I lost 30 pounds," says Gale. "He took me on a romantic weekend to the mountains. It was wonderful. And I was able to ski again, without feeling clumsy and fat."

Jay lost 40 pounds after giving up a diet of French fries, pizzas, hoagies and ice cream. He lost five inches from his waist alone.

(Continued on page 200)

1,000-CALORIE PLAN*
Week 1
5% Calories from Fat

Breakfast		Lunch		Dinner	
SUNDAY					
1 cup apple juice	116	½ cup low-fat cottage cheese	82	Mollen's Mushroom Omelet	97
1 cup oatmeal with	146	Relish plate:		Mixed salad:	
1 cup skim milk	88	1 medium tomato, sliced	33	2 cups shredded lettuce	20
1 medium banana	101	½ cup sliced green peppers	17	1 cup sliced celery	20
	451	1 medium carrot, sliced	30	½ cup sliced radishes	10
		2 tablespoons Buttermilk Dressing	12	2 tablespoons Italian Dressing	5
		½ cup grape juice	84	1 slice whole wheat bread with	61
			258	1 tablespoon apple butter	37
				1 small apple	58
					308

Total calories: 1,017

Breakfast		Lunch		Dinner	
MONDAY					
Mollen Milkshake	350	Tuna salad:		Vegetable platter:	
1 slice rye toast	61	2 ounces water-packed tuna	72	¼ cup low-fat cottage cheese	41
	411	1 medium tomato, wedged	33	½ cup broccoli flowerets	20
		½ cup sliced celery	10	½ cup cauliflower flowerets	14
		½ cup sliced cucumbers	8	1 medium carrot, julienned	30
		2 cups shredded lettuce	20	½ cup sliced green peppers	17

2 tablespoons *Mustard Dressing* — 134

2 rye wafers	18
1 medium apple	45
1 cup skim milk	87
	88
	381

1 cup peach nectar — 256

Total calories: 1,048

TUESDAY

½ cup orange juice	56
½ medium grapefruit	41
1 whole wheat English muffin with	140
2 teaspoons fruit preserves	37
1 cup skim milk	88
	362

Toasted cheese sandwich: Broil

1 slice lightly toasted whole wheat bread topped with	61
1 ounce part-skim American cheese, sliced	90
1 medium tomato	33
1 medium apple	87
	271

1 serving *Fish and Vegetables à l'Orange*	188
1 small baked potato with	90
2 tablespoons *Mollenized Sour Cream*	24
1 slice whole wheat bread	61
¾ cup strawberries, sliced	33
	396

Total calories: 1,029

WEDNESDAY

½ cup apple juice	58
½ medium banana	50
½ cup Grape-Nuts with	202
1 cup skim milk	88
	398

Spinach salad:

2 cups shredded spinach	28
½ cup sliced mushrooms	10
½ cup sliced beets	27
½ cup bean sprouts	23
½ cup zucchini strips	11
2 tablespoons *Mustard Dressing*	18
4 rye wafers	90
1 small apple	58
	265

3 ounces cod, baked, broiled or poached	140
1 serving *Cheesy Potatoes*	190
½ cup steamed broccoli with	20
2 tablespoons *Buttermilk Dressing*	12
	362

Total calories: 1,025

*Recipes for italicized dishes begin on page 237. Recipes are arranged according to alphabetical order for easy reference.

(Continued)

1,000-CALORIE PLAN–*Continued*
Week 1

Breakfast		Lunch		Dinner	
THURSDAY					
½ medium banana	50	1 cup *Cucumber Soup*	55	1 *Vegetable Kabob*	125
2 biscuits Shredded Wheat with	166	2 slices pumpernickel bread	158	1 serving *Rice Pilaf*	247
1 cup skim milk	88	1 small apple	58	1 medium navel orange	65
	304		271		437
Total calories: 1,012					
FRIDAY					
½ cup orange juice	56	*Mollen Milkshake*	350	1 cup cooked spaghetti with	192
2 servings *Cottage Cheese and Cinnamon Toast*	204	1 small apple	58	½ cup tomato sauce and	35
1 cup skim milk	88		408	½ cup cooked sliced mushrooms	10
	348			Mixed salad:	
				1 cup shredded lettuce	10
				½ cup sliced radishes	10
				½ cup sliced cucumbers	8
				2 tablespoons *Italian Dressing*	5
					270
Total calories: 1,026					

SATURDAY

Breakfast		Lunch		Dinner	
½ cup grape juice	84	Fruit salad:		1 serving *Low-Fat Spinach Bake*	166
2 slices whole wheat toast with	122	1 small apple, diced	58	1 small baked potato with	90
2 teaspoons fruit preserves	37	1 medium navel orange, diced	65	2 tablespoons *Mollenized Sour Cream*	24
1 cup skim milk	88	1 medium banana, sliced	101	1 whole wheat dinner roll	70
	331	1 medium peach, sliced	38	1 cup strawberries, sliced	44
		¼ cup *Fruit Salad Dressing*	32		394
			294		

Total calories 1,019

Week 2
10% Calories from Fat

SUNDAY

Breakfast		Lunch		Dinner	
½ medium cantaloupe	94	1 *Fruit Blintze*	70	1 serving *Tart and Creamy Coleslaw*	24
¾ cup 40% Bran Flakes with	110	2 slices melba toast	30	3 ounces pink salmon,* baked, broiled or poached	120
½ cup skim milk	44	½ cup low-fat cottage cheese with	82	½ cup steamed broccoli	20
1 slice whole wheat toast with	61	1 medium tomato, wedged	33	1 serving *Stuffed Potatoes*	70
1 tablespoon apple butter	37	1 small apple	58	1 whole wheat dinner roll with	70
	346	herbal tea with lemon wedge	5	1 teaspoon margarine	34
			278	15 large sweet cherries	70
					408

Total calories: 1,032

*Chinook and sockeye have a higher fat and calorie content.

(Continued)

1,000-CALORIE PLAN–Continued
Week 2

	Breakfast		Lunch		Dinner

MONDAY

	Breakfast		Lunch		Dinner
½ cup orange juice	56	1 cup clear vegetable soup	64	1 serving *Cucumber-Onion Salad*	27
2 slices French toast made with		1 slice rye bread	61	1 serving *Hearty Halibut*	150
2 slices whole wheat bread	122	1 ounce part-skim American		1 medium carrot, sliced and	30
1 egg	78	cheese, sliced	90	steamed	
1 tablespoon skim milk	5	1 medium apple	87	1 serving *Pears in Wine*	90
nonstick vegetable spray	0		302		297
Topped with					
2 teaspoons fruit preserves	37				
1 cup skim milk	88				
	386				

Total calories: 985

TUESDAY

	Breakfast		Lunch		Dinner
½ cup pineapple juice	70	*Mollen Milkshake*	350	1 serving *Stuffed Celery*	13
½ cup Raisin Bran with	84	1 medium apple	87	1 serving *Poached Chicken Breast*	150
1 cup skim milk	88		437	1 serving *Tangy Cauliflower*	27
1 medium navel orange	65			1 slice whole wheat bread	61
	307				251

Total calories: 995

WEDNESDAY

½ cup grape juice	84
1 slice raisin toast with	70
1 teaspoon margarine and a sprinkle of cinnamon	34
	0
1 cup skim milk	88
	276

⅔ cup tomato juice	34
1 ounce part-skim mozzarella cheese, cubed	72
6 whole wheat crackers	174
1 large apple, wedged	133
	413

1 serving *Triple Bean Salad*	61
1 serving *Red Snapper*	113
1 serving *Orangey Carrots*	37
1 slice whole wheat bread	61
1 medium peach	38
	310

Total calories: 999

THURSDAY

1 cup grapefruit juice	96
½ cup All-Bran with	107
1 cup skim milk	88
	291

Relish plate:	
1 medium carrot, julienned	30
1 large stalk celery, julienned	9
2 tablespoons *Buttermilk Dressing*	12
2 large graham crackers with	110
2 tablespoons *Mollenized Sour Cream*	24
1 large pear	122
1 cup club soda with lime wedge	0
	307

2 *Stuffed Mushrooms*	22
1 serving *Oriental Chicken*	205
½ cup cooked brown rice	116
1 medium apple	87
	430

Total calories: 1,028

FRIDAY

¼ honeydew melon	116
1 serving *Cottage Cheese and Cinnamon Toast*	102
1 cup skim milk	88
	306

Cottage cheese and fresh fruit plate:	
½ cup low-fat cottage cheese	82
1 medium apple, wedged	87
½ cup strawberries, sliced	22
2 medium prunes, sliced	41
1 medium navel orange, wedged	65
3 slices melba toast	45
	342

3 ounces cod, baked, broiled or poached	140
1 cup steamed cauliflower	28
1 whole wheat dinner roll with	70
1 teaspoon margarine	34
1 serving *Fruit Ambrosia*	60
	332

Total calories: 980

(Continued)

1,000-CALORIE PLAN – Continued
Week 2

Breakfast	Lunch	Dinner
SATURDAY		
½ cup orange juice 56	Yogurt-pineapple refresher:	Tuna melt:
½ cup Grape-Nuts with 202	1 cup plain, low-fat yogurt mixed with 144	Broil
1 cup skim milk 88	½ cup crushed pineapple packed in its own juice and 75	1 slice lightly toasted whole wheat bread topped with 61
346	2 tablespoons raisins 62	2 ounces water-packed tuna and 72
	herbal tea with lemon wedge 5	1 ounce part-skim American cheese, shredded 70
	286	1 small apple 58
		1 12-ounce light beer 95
		356

Total calories: 988

Week 3
15% Calories from Fat

Breakfast	Lunch	Dinner
SUNDAY		
1 medium banana 101	Tossed tuna salad:	1 serving *Marinated Vegetables* 23
1 cup All-Bran with 214	2 ounces water-packed tuna 72	1 cup cooked spaghetti with 192
1 cup skim milk 88	1 cup shredded romaine lettuce 10	½ cup tomato sauce 35
403		

1 cup shredded red-leaf lettuce	10
½ medium cucumber, sliced	15
1 ounce low-fat string cheese, shredded	90
2 tablespoons *Mustard Dressing*	18
2 slices melba toast	30
1 small apple	58
	303

Dinner salad:

1 cup shredded lettuce	10
¼ cup croutons	14
2 tablespoons *Italian Dressing*	5
	279

Total calories: 985

MONDAY

½ cup orange juice	56
½ cup oatmeal with	73
2 tablespoons raisins and	62
½ cup skim milk	44
1 small apple	58
	293

Cheese crisps:
Broil

2 12-inch tortillas sprinkled with	252
1 ounce part-skim American cheese, shredded	90
1 *Banana Pop*	60
	402

1 serving *Marinated Halibut*	144
1 serving *Asparagus Delight*	16
1 serving *Parslied Potatoes*	66
1 serving *Carrot-Orange Toss*	100
	326

Total calories: 1,021

TUESDAY

½ cup apple juice	58
1 whole wheat English muffin with	140
1 teaspoon peanut butter	32
1 cup skim milk	88
	318

Cucumber boat:

1 medium cucumber stuffed with	30
2 ounces water-packed tuna	72
2 slices whole wheat bread	122
1 small apple	58
1 cup *Sparkling Juice* (grape)	84
	366

1 *Chicken Kabob* (appetizer)	34
1 serving *Spinach Casserole*	203
1 small baked potato with	90
1 tablespoon *Mollenized Sour Cream*	12
	339

Total calories: 1,023

(Continued)

1,000-CALORIE PLAN – Continued
Week 3

Breakfast	Lunch	Dinner
WEDNESDAY		
1 cup mixed juice:	1 serving *Turkey Chili* 155	1 serving *Sole with Yogurt Sauce* 124
½ cup pineapple juice mixed with 70	Tossed salad:	1 serving *Mashed Squash* 61
½ cup grapefruit juice 48	1 cup shredded romaine lettuce 10	1 slice whole wheat bread 61
2 biscuits Shredded Wheat with 166	1 cup shredded red-leaf lettuce 10	1 serving *Ambrosia Medley* 95
1 cup skim milk 88	½ medium tomato, sliced 16	341
1 small apple 58	⅛ avocado, sliced 45	
430	2 tablespoons *Italian Dressing* 5	
	241	
Total calories: 1,012		
THURSDAY		
¾ cup peach nectar 101	1 cup chicken consommé 39	⅔ cup vegetable juice 34
½ cup All-Bran with 107	Fruit salad:	1 serving *Sole and Broccoli with Rice* 268
1 cup skim milk 88	1 medium apple, sliced 87	1 cup strawberries, sliced 44
296	1 medium navel orange, sliced 65	346
	1 medium banana, sliced 101	
	½ cup *Fruit Salad Dressing* 64	
	356	
Total calories: 998		

FRIDAY

½ cup prune juice	92
1 *Mollen Muffin*	103
1 cup skim milk	88
	283

Peanut butter and banana sandwich:	
2 slices whole wheat bread	122
2 teaspoons peanut butter	64
1 small banana, sliced	85
1 cup grapes	53
	324

Mollen Milkshake	350
1 small apple	58
	408

Total calories: 1,015

SATURDAY

1 medium banana	101
½ cup Grape-Nuts with	202
1 cup skim milk	88
	391

Health salad:	
2 cups shredded lettuce	20
½ cup sliced cucumbers	8
½ medium tomato, sliced	16
1 small apple, diced	58
1 tablespoon sunflower seeds	45
1 ounce low-fat string cheese, shredded	90
2 tablespoons *Buttermilk Dressing*	12
2 rye wafers	45
	294

⅔ cup tomato juice	34
½ chicken breast, baked, broiled or poached	145
¾ cup steamed green beans with	25
½ cup cooked sliced mushrooms	10
½ cup mashed potatoes with	70
1 teaspoon margarine	34
	318

Total calories: 1,003

(Continued)

1,000-CALORIE PLAN – Continued
Week 4
20% Calories from Fat

Breakfast		Lunch		Dinner	
SUNDAY					
½ cup orange juice	56	1 serving *Lean Lasagna*	275	1 serving *Patio Potato Salad*	103
1 serving *Whole Wheat Bran Pancakes* with	138	Tossed salad:		3 *Chicken Kabobs*	102
1 tablespoon apple butter	37	1 cup shredded lettuce	10	1 cup *Spicy Lemon Iced Tea*	64
1 cup skim milk	88	½ medium tomato, sliced	16		269
	319	2 tablespoons *Italian Dressing*	5		
		1 serving *Art's Brown Apple*	140		
			446		
Total calories: 1,034					
MONDAY					
½ cup apple juice	58	1 serving *Stuffed Tomato Salad*	128	1 serving *Orange-Carrot Salad*	49
2 biscuits *Shredded Wheat* with	166	6 slices melba toast	90	1 serving *Sole Florentine*	130
1 cup skim milk	88	1 small apple	58	1 small baked potato with	90
	312	½ cup grape juice	84	2 tablespoons *Mollenized Sour Cream*	24
			360	1 medium navel orange	65
					358
Total calories: 1,030					

TUESDAY

½ cup grapefruit juice	48
1 cup strawberries, sliced	44
2 slices whole wheat toast with	122
1 teaspoon margarine	34
1 cup skim milk	88
	336

2 cups *Cucumber Soup*	110
1 slice pumpernickel bread with	79
1 teaspoon margarine	34
1 medium apple	87
	310

3 ounces baked turkey breast fillets	115
2 servings *Spinach Royale*	60
1 medium banana	101
1 medium orange	65
	341

Total calories: 987

WEDNESDAY

⅓ papaya, sliced	39
½ cup oatmeal with	73
1 tablespoon raisins and	31
1 cup skim milk	88
	231

1 serving *Tangy Chicken Salad*	230
on a bed of lettuce	15
1 *Pineapple Pop*	90
	335

1 serving *Waldorf Salad*	110
1 serving *Fish Creole*	238
½ cup steamed brussels sprouts	28
1 slice pumpernickel bread	79
	455

Total calories: 1,021

THURSDAY

½ cup apricot nectar	71
1 serving *Whole Wheat Bran Pancakes* with	138
1 tablespoon fruit preserves	56
1 cup skim milk	88
	353

1 *Chicken Pocket Sandwich*	284
1½ cups plain popcorn (air popped)	35
1 cup club soda with lime wedge	0
	319

1 *Chilled Shrimp and Mushroom Kabob*	200
1 serving *Pineapple Baked Apple*	160
	360

Total calories: 1,032

(Continued)

1,000-CALORIE PLAN – Continued
Week 4

	Breakfast		Lunch		Dinner	
FRIDAY						
	1 slice whole wheat toast with	61	1 serving Turkey-Squash Bake	230	Dr. Art's Avocado Omelet	157
	1 teaspoon margarine	34	1 serving Fruit Slush	60	1 whole wheat English muffin with	140
	½ cup All-Bran with	107		290	1 teaspoon margarine	34
	1 cup skim milk	88			¾ cup diced fresh pineapple	52
	1 small apple	58				383
		348				

Total calories: 1,021

	Breakfast		Lunch		Dinner	
SATURDAY						
	¾ cup pear nectar	94	1 serving Fish and Vegetables à		1 serving Saucy Chicken and	
	1 Mollen Muffin with	103	l'Orange	188	Cheese	190
	1 tablespoon honey	64	1 medium ear corn on the cob with	70	½ cup steamed eggplant	19
	1 cup skim milk	88	1 teaspoon margarine	34	1 slice whole wheat bread with	61
		349	1 medium apple	87	1 teaspoon margarine	34
				379		304

Total calories: 1,032

1,500-CALORIE PLAN*
Week 1
5% Calories from Fat

Breakfast		Lunch		Dinner	
SUNDAY					
1 cup apple juice	116	1 cup low-fat cottage cheese	164	*Mollen's Mushroom Omelet*	97
1 medium banana	101	Relish plate:		Mixed salad:	
1 cup oatmeal with	146	1 medium tomato, sliced	33	2 cups shredded lettuce	20
1 cup skim milk	88	½ cup sliced green peppers	17	1 cup sliced celery	20
	——	1 medium carrot, sliced	30	½ cup sliced radishes	10
	451	2 tablespoons *Buttermilk Dressing*	12	2 tablespoons *Italian Dressing*	5
		6 rye wafers	135	2 slices whole wheat bread with	122
		½ cup grape juice	84	2 tablespoons apple butter	74
			——	1 large apple	133
			475	1 cup skim milk	88
					——
					569

Total calories: 1,495

*Recipes for italicized dishes begin on page 237. Recipes are arranged according to alphabetical order for easy reference.

(Continued)

1,500-CALORIE PLAN – Continued
Week 1

Breakfast	Lunch	Dinner

MONDAY

Breakfast		Lunch		Dinner	
Mollen Milkshake	350	Tuna salad:		½ cup orange juice	56
2 slices rye bread with	122	3 ounces water-packed tuna	108	Vegetable platter:	
2 tablespoons fruit preserves	108	1 medium tomato, sliced	33	½ cup low-fat cottage cheese	82
	580	½ cup sliced celery	10	½ cup broccoli flowerets	20
		½ cup sliced cucumbers	8	½ cup cauliflower flowerets	14
		2 cups shredded lettuce	20	1 large carrot, julienned	42
		2 tablespoons *Mustard Dressing*	18	½ cup sliced green peppers	17
		4 slices melba toast	60	2 slices pumpernickel bread	158
		1 large apple	133	1 cup skim milk	88
		1 cup skim milk	88		477
			478		

Total calories: 1,535

TUESDAY

Breakfast		Lunch		Dinner	
1 cup orange juice	112	Toasted cheese sandwich:		1 serving *Fish and Vegetables à l'Orange*	188
½ medium grapefruit	41	Broil		1 medium baked potato with	145
1 whole wheat English muffin with	140	2 slices lightly toasted whole wheat bread topped with	122	2 tablespoons *Mollenized Sour Cream*	24
1 tablespoon fruit preserves	54	1 ounce part-skim American cheese, sliced	90	2 slices whole wheat bread with	122
1 cup skim milk	88			2 tablespoons apple butter	74
	435				

		1 cup strawberries, sliced	44
			597
1 medium tomato	33		
1 large apple	133		
1 cup skim milk	88		
	466		

Total calories: 1,498

WEDNESDAY

½ cup apple juice	58				
1 medium banana	101				
½ cup Grape-Nuts with	202				
1 cup skim milk	88				
	449				
Spinach salad:				4 ounces cod, baked, broiled or poached	186
2 cups shredded spinach		28		1 serving *Cheesy Potatoes*	190
½ cup sliced mushrooms		10		½ cup steamed broccoli with	20
½ cup sliced beets		27		2 tablespoons *Buttermilk Dressing*	12
½ cup bean sprouts		23		1 medium apple	87
½ cup zucchini strips		11		1 cup skim milk	88
2 tablespoons *Mustard Dressing*		18			583
10 rye wafers		225			
1 cup pear nectar		125			
		467			

Total calories: 1,499

THURSDAY

½ cup grape juice	84				
1 medium banana	101				
3 biscuits Shredded Wheat with	249				
1 cup skim milk	88				
	522				
2 cups *Cucumber Soup*		110		2 *Vegetable Kabobs*	250
½ cup low-fat cottage cheese		82		1 serving *Rice Pilaf*	247
1 slice pumpernickel bread		79		1 medium navel orange	65
1 medium apple		87		1 cup skim milk	88
		358			650

Total calories: 1,530

(Continued)

1,500-CALORIE PLAN – Continued
Week 1

Breakfast		Lunch		Dinner	
FRIDAY					
1 cup orange juice	112	*Mollen Milkshake*	350	1 cup cooked spaghetti with	192
2 servings *Cottage Cheese and Cinnamon Toast*	204	10 rye wafers	225	½ cup tomato sauce and	35
1 cup skim milk	88	1 large apple	133	½ cup cooked sliced mushrooms	10
	404		708	Mixed salad:	
				1 cup shredded lettuce	10
				½ cup sliced radishes	10
				½ cup sliced cucumbers	8
				2 tablespoons *Italian Dressing*	5
				1 cup grapes	53
				1 cup skim milk	88
					411
Total calories: 1,523					
SATURDAY					
1 cup orange juice	112	Fruit salad:		1 serving *Low-Fat Spinach Bake*	166
2 slices whole wheat toast with	122	½ cup low-fat cottage cheese	82	1 medium baked potato with	145
2 tablespoons fruit preserves	108	1 medium apple, diced	87	2 tablespoons *Mollenized Sour Cream*	24
1 cup skim milk	88	1 medium navel orange, diced	65	2 slices pumpernickel bread	158
	430	1 medium banana, sliced	101	1 cup strawberries, sliced	44
		¼ cup *Fruit Salad Dressing*	32		537
		6 slices melba toast	90		
		1 cup skim milk	88		
			545		
Total calories: 1,512					

Week 2
10% Calories from Fat

Breakfast		Lunch		Dinner	
SUNDAY					
¼ medium cantaloupe	47	1 cup chicken consommé	39	1 serving *Tart and Creamy Coleslaw*	24
1 cup 40% Bran Flakes with	146	2 *Fruit Blintzes*	140	4 ounces pink salmon,* baked, broiled or poached	160
1 cup skim milk	88	6 slices melba toast	90	1 cup steamed broccoli	40
1 slice whole wheat toast with	61	½ cup low-fat cottage cheese with	82	2 servings *Stuffed Potatoes*	140
1 tablespoon apple butter	37	1 medium tomato, wedged	33	2 whole wheat dinner rolls with	140
		herbal tea with lemon wedge	5	1 teaspoon margarine	34
	379		389	1 large apple	133
				1 cup skim milk	88
					759

Total calories: 1,527

*Chinook and sockeye have a higher fat and calorie content.

Breakfast		Lunch		Dinner	
MONDAY					
1 cup orange juice	112	1 cup clear vegetable soup	64	1 serving *Cucumber-Onion Salad*	27
2 slices French toast made with		2 slices rye bread	122	1½ servings *Hearty Halibut*	225
2 slices whole wheat bread	122	1 ounce part-skim American cheese, sliced	90	2 medium carrots, sliced and steamed	60
1 egg	78	1 large apple	133	2 servings *Pears in Wine*	180
1 tablespoon skim milk	5		409	1 cup skim milk	88
nonstick vegetable spray	0				580
Topped with					
2 tablespoons fruit preserves	108				
1 cup skim milk	88				
	513				

Total calories: 1,502

(Continued)

1,500-CALORIE PLAN – Continued
Week 2

Breakfast		Lunch		Dinner	
TUESDAY					
½ cup pineapple juice	70	*Mollen Milkshake*	350	4 servings *Stuffed Celery*	52
1 cup Raisin Bran with	168	4 rye wafers	90	1 serving *Poached Chicken Breast*	150
1 cup skim milk	88	1 large apple	133	2 servings *Tangy Cauliflower*	54
1 slice whole wheat toast with	61		573	2 slices whole wheat bread	122
1 tablespoon apple butter	37			½ cup juice-packed sliced peaches	29
	424			1 cup skim milk	88
					495
Total calories: 1,492					
WEDNESDAY					
1 cup orange juice	112	⅔ cup tomato juice	34	2 servings *Triple Bean Salad*	122
¼ medium cantaloupe	47	1 cup low-fat cottage cheese	164	1½ servings *Red Snapper*	170
2 slices raisin toast with	140	8 whole wheat crackers	232	2 servings *Orangey Carrots*	74
1 teaspoon margarine and a	34	1 large apple, wedged	133	1 slice whole wheat bread	61
sprinkle of cinnamon	0		563	1 cup skim milk	88
1 cup skim milk	88				515
	421				
Total calories: 1,499					

THURSDAY

1 cup grapefruit juice	96
1 cup blueberries	82
1 cup 40% Bran Flakes with	146
1 cup skim milk	88
	412

Relish plate:	
1 medium carrot, julienned	30
1 large stalk celery, julienned	9
2 tablespoons *Buttermilk Dressing*	12
3 large graham crackers with	165
2 tablespoons *Mollenized Sour Cream*	24
1 large pear	122
1 cup club soda with lime wedge	0
	362

4 *Stuffed Mushrooms*	44
1 serving *Oriental Chicken*	205
½ cup cooked brown rice	116
2 slices whole wheat bread with	122
1 tablespoon apple butter	37
1 large apple	133
1 cup skim milk	88
	745

Total calories: 1,519

FRIDAY

½ cup orange juice	56
¼ medium honeydew melon	116
2 servings *Cottage Cheese and Cinnamon Toast*	204
1 cup skim milk	88
	464

Cottage cheese and fresh fruit plate:	
½ cup low-fat cottage cheese	82
1 large apple, wedged	133
4 medium prunes, sliced	82
1 medium navel orange, wedged	65
6 slices melba toast	90
1 cup skim milk	88
	540

1 cup clear vegetable soup	64
4 ounces cod, baked, broiled or poached	186
1 cup steamed cauliflower	28
1 whole wheat dinner roll with	70
1 teaspoon margarine	34
2 servings *Fruit Ambrosia*	120
	502

Total calories: 1,506

(Continued)

1,500-CALORIE PLAN – *Continued*
Week 2

	Breakfast	Lunch	Dinner
SATURDAY			
1 cup orange juice	112	Yogurt-pineapple refresher:		Tuna melt:	
1 slice whole wheat toast	61	1 cup plain, low-fat yogurt, mixed with	144	Broil	
½ cup Grape-Nuts with	202	¾ cup crushed pineapple packed in its own juice and	113	2 slices lightly toasted whole wheat bread topped with	122
1 cup skim milk	88			3 ounces water-packed tuna and	108
	463	2 tablespoons raisins	62	1 ounce part-skim American cheese, shredded	70
		8 rye wafers	180	1 large apple	133
		herbal tea with lemon wedge	5	1 12-ounce light beer	95
			504		528

Total calories: 1,495

Week 3
15% Calories from Fat

	Breakfast	Lunch	Dinner
SUNDAY			
1 cup orange juice	112	Tossed tuna salad:		1 serving *Marinated Vegetables*	23
1 medium banana	101	4 ounces water-packed tuna	144	1 cup cooked spaghetti with	192

Item	Calories
1 cup All-Bran with	214
1 cup skim milk	88
	515

Item	Calories
1 cup shredded romaine lettuce	10
1 cup shredded red-leaf lettuce	10
1 medium tomato, wedged	33
½ medium cucumber, sliced	15
1 ounce low-fat string cheese, shredded	90
2 tablespoons *Mustard Dressing*	18
3 rye wafers	67
1 large apple	133
1 cup skim milk	88
	608

Item	Calories
½ cup tomato sauce	35
Dinner salad:	
2 cups shredded lettuce	20
¼ cup croutons	14
2 tablespoons *Italian Dressing*	5
1 slice whole wheat bread with	61
1 teaspoon margarine	34
	384

Total calories: 1,507

MONDAY

Item	Calories
½ cup apple juice	58
1 cup oatmeal with	146
2 tablespoons raisins and	62
1 cup skim milk	88
	354

Item	Calories
Cheese crisps:	
Broil	
2 12-inch tortillas sprinkled with	252
1 ounce part-skim American cheese, shredded	90
1 *Banana Pop*	60
1 medium navel orange	65
1 cup skim milk	88
	555

Item	Calories
1½ servings *Marinated Halibut*	216
2 servings *Asparagus Delight*	32
2 servings *Parslied Potatoes*	132
1 slice whole wheat bread with	61
1 teaspoon margarine	34
1 large apple	133
	608

Total calories: 1,517

(Continued)

1,500-CALORIE PLAN – Continued
Week 3

Breakfast		Lunch		Dinner	
TUESDAY					
1 cup apple juice	116	Cucumber boat:		1 Chicken Kabob (appetizer)	34
2 whole wheat English muffins with	280	1 medium cucumber stuffed	30	1 serving Spinach Casserole	203
2 teaspoons peanut butter	64	with		1 medium baked potato with	145
1 cup skim milk	88	3 ounces water-packed tuna	108	2 tablespoons Mollenized Sour	
	——	2 slices whole wheat bread with	122	Cream	24
	548	1 teaspoon margarine	34	1 cup skim milk	88
		1 medium apple	87		——
		1 cup Sparkling Juice (grape)	84		494
			——		
			465		
Total calories: 1,507					
WEDNESDAY					
1 cup mixed juice:		1 serving Turkey Chili	155	1½ servings Sole with Yogurt Sauce	186
½ cup pineapple juice mixed	70	Tossed salad:		2 servings Mashed Squash	122
with		1 cup shredded romaine		1 serving Ambrosia Medley	95
½ cup grapefruit juice	48	lettuce	10	1 whole wheat dinner roll	70
3 biscuits Shredded Wheat with	249	1 cup shredded red-leaf		1 medium navel orange	65
1 cup skim milk	88	lettuce	10		——
	——	2 medium tomatoes, sliced	64		538
	455	⅛ avocado, sliced	45		
		2 tablespoons Italian			
		Dressing	5		
		1 large apple	133		
		1 cup skim milk	88		
			——		
			510		
Total calories: 1,503					

THURSDAY

¾ cup peach nectar	101
½ cup All-Bran with	107
2 tablespoons raisins and	62
1 cup skim milk	88
	358

Fruit salad:

1 large apple, sliced	133
1 medium navel orange, sliced	65
1 medium banana, sliced	101
½ cup *Fruit Salad Dressing*	64
4 slices melba toast	60
1 cup skim milk	88
	511

⅔ cup vegetable juice	34
1½ servings *Sole and Broccoli with Rice*	402
2 slices whole wheat bread with	122
1 teaspoon margarine	34
1 cup strawberries, sliced	44
	636

Total calories: 1,505

FRIDAY

¾ cup prune juice	138
1 *Mollen Muffin* with	103
1 tablespoon honey	64
1 cup skim milk	88
	393

Peanut butter and banana sandwich:

2 slices whole wheat bread	122
2 teaspoons peanut butter	64
1 small banana, sliced	85
1 large apple	133
1 cup skim milk	88
	492

Mollen Milkshake	350
4 ounces baked turkey breast fillets	153
2 slices rye bread	122
	625

Total calories: 1,510

(Continued)

1,500-CALORIE PLAN—*Continued*
Week 3

Breakfast	Lunch	Dinner
SATURDAY		
1 cup orange juice — 112	Health salad:	⅔ cup tomato juice — 34
¾ cup Grape-Nuts with — 303	2 cups shredded lettuce — 20	1 serving *Poached Chicken Breast* — 150
1 medium banana, sliced, and — 101	½ cup sliced cucumbers — 8	¾ cup steamed green beans with — 25
1 cup skim milk — 88	1 medium tomato, sliced — 32	½ cup cooked sliced
	1 medium apple, diced — 87	mushrooms — 10
604	1 tablespoon sunflower seeds — 45	½ cup mashed potatoes with — 70
	1 ounce low-fat string	1 teaspoon margarine — 34
	cheese, shredded — 90	1 medium peach — 38
	2 tablespoons *Buttermilk*	1 12-ounce light beer — 95
	Dressing — 12	456
	6 slices melba toast — 90	
	1 cup skim milk — 88	
	472	

Total calories: 1,532

Week 4
20% Calories from Fat

Breakfast		Lunch		Dinner	
SUNDAY					
1 cup orange juice	112	1 serving *Lean Lasagna*	275	1 serving *Patio Potato Salad*	103
1 serving *Whole Wheat Bran*		Tossed salad:		4 *Chicken Kabobs*	136
Pancakes with	138	2 cups shredded lettuce	20	1 whole wheat dinner roll with	70
2 teaspoons peanut butter and	64	1 medium tomato, wedged	32	1 teaspoon margarine	34
1 tablespoon apple butter	37	2 tablespoons *Italian Dressing*	5	1 medium navel orange	65
1 cup skim milk	88	1 serving *Art's Brown Apple*	140	1 cup *Spicy Lemon Iced Tea*	64
	439	1 cup skim milk	88		472
			560		
Total calories: 1,471					
MONDAY					
1 cup grapefruit juice	96	2 servings *Stuffed Tomato Salad*	256	2 servings *Orange-Carrot Salad*	98
3 biscuits Shredded Wheat with	249	4 rye wafers	90	1½ servings *Sole Florentine*	195
1 cup skim milk	88	1 large apple	133	1 small baked potato with	90
	433		479	2 tablespoons *Mollenized*	
				Sour Cream	24
				1 slice whole wheat bread	61
				1 medium navel orange	65
				1 cup skim milk	88
					621
Total calories: 1,533					

(Continued)

1,500-CALORIE PLAN – Continued
Week 4

Breakfast		Lunch		Dinner	

TUESDAY

Breakfast		Lunch		Dinner	
1 cup grapefruit juice	96	⅔ cup tomato juice	34	1 serving *Waldorf Salad*	110
1 cup strawberries, sliced	44	1 serving *Tangy Chicken Salad*	230	1 serving *Fish Creole*	238
2 slices whole wheat toast with	122	on a bed of lettuce	15	½ cup steamed brussels sprouts	28
1 teaspoon margarine	34	6 slices melba toast	90	2 slices pumpernickel bread with	158
1 cup skim milk	88	1 *Pineapple Pop*	90	1 teaspoon margarine	34
				1 cup skim milk	88
	384		459		656

Total calories: 1,499

WEDNESDAY

Breakfast		Lunch		Dinner	
½ papaya	58	2 cups *Cucumber Soup*	110	4 ounces baked turkey breast fillets	153
1 cup oatmeal with	146	2 slices whole wheat bread with	122	2 servings *Spinach Royale*	60
2 tablespoons raisins and	62	2 teaspoons margarine	68	1 medium baked potato with	145
1 cup skim milk	88	1 large apple	133	2 tablespoons *Mollenized Sour*	24
		1 cup skim milk	88	*Cream*	
				1 medium banana	101
				1 cup orange juice	112
	354		521		595

Total calories: 1,470

THURSDAY

¾ cup apricot nectar	107
1 serving *Whole Wheat Bran Pancakes* with	138
2 tablespoons fruit preserves	108
1 cup skim milk	88
1 small apple	58
	499
1 *Chicken Pocket Sandwich*	284
3 cups plain popcorn (air popped)	70
1 medium banana	101
1 cup club soda with lime wedge	0
	455
1 *Chilled Shrimp and Mushroom Kabob*	200
1 cup cooked brown rice	116
½ serving *Pineapple Baked Apple*	160
1 cup skim milk	88
	564

Total calories: 1,518

FRIDAY

½ medium grapefruit	41
2 slices whole wheat toast with	122
2 teaspoons peanut butter	64
1 cup skim milk	88
	315
1 serving *Turkey-Squash Bake*	230
1 cup low-fat cottage cheese	164
6 slices melba toast	90
1 large apple	133
1 serving *Fruit Slush*	60
	677
Dr. Art's Avocado Omelet	157
1 whole wheat English muffin with	140
1 teaspoon margarine	34
1 cup diced fresh pineapple	69
1 cup skim milk	88
	488

Total calories: 1,480

SATURDAY

¾ cup pear nectar	94
2 *Mollen Muffins* with	206
1 tablespoon honey	64
1 cup skim milk	88
	452
1 serving *Fish and Vegetables à l'Orange*	188
1 medium ear corn on the cob with	70
1 teaspoon margarine	34
1 cup juice-packed fruit cocktail	74
½ cup grape juice	84
	450
1 serving *Saucy Chicken and Cheese*	190
1 cup steamed eggplant	38
2 slices whole wheat bread with	122
1 teaspoon margarine	34
1 large apple	133
1 cup skim milk	88
	605

Total calories: 1,507

(Continued)

2,000-CALORIE PLAN*
Week 1
5% Calories from Fat

Breakfast		Lunch		Dinner	
SUNDAY					
1 cup apple juice	116	½ cup grapefruit juice	48	*Mollen's Mushroom Omelet*	97
1 medium banana	101	1 cup low-fat cottage cheese	164	Mixed salad:	
1½ cups oatmeal with	219	Relish plate:		2 cups shredded lettuce	20
2 tablespoons raisins and	62	1 medium tomato, sliced	33	1 cup sliced celery	20
1 cup skim milk	88	1 cup sliced green peppers	34	½ cup sliced radishes	10
	___	2 medium carrots, julienned	60	2 tablespoons *Italian Dressing*	5
	586	2 tablespoons *Buttermilk*		3 slices whole wheat bread with	183
		Dressing	12	2 tablespoons apple butter	74
		4 rye wafers	90	1 large apple	133
		1 large apple	133	1 medium navel orange	65
		1 medium navel orange	65	1 cup skim milk	88
		1 cup skim milk	88		___
			___		695
			727		
Total calories: 2,008					
MONDAY					
Mollen Milkshake	350	1 cup orange juice	112	¾ cup peach nectar	101
3 slices rye bread with	183	Tuna salad:		Vegetable platter:	
2 tablespoons fruit preserves	108	3 ounces water-packed tuna	108	½ cup low-fat cottage cheese	82
	___	1 medium tomato, sliced	33	1 cup broccoli flowerets	40
	641				

MONDAY *(continued)*

Item	Calories
½ cup sliced celery	10
½ cup sliced cucumbers	8
2 cups shredded lettuce	20
2 tablespoons *Mustard Dressing*	18
6 whole wheat crackers	174
1 large apple	133
1 cup skim milk	88
	704

Item	Calories
1 cup cauliflower flowerets	28
2 medium carrots, sliced	60
½ cup sliced green peppers	17
2 slices pumpernickel bread	158
1 large apple	133
1 cup skim milk	88
	707

Total calories: 2,052

TUESDAY

Item	Calories
1 cup orange juice	112
½ medium grapefruit	41
2 whole wheat English muffins with	280
2 tablespoons fruit preserves	108
1 cup skim milk	88
	629

Item	Calories
Toasted cheese sandwich:	
Broil	
2 slices lightly toasted whole wheat bread topped with	122
2 ounces part-skim American cheese, sliced	180
1 medium tomato	33
1 large apple	133
1 cup skim milk	88
	556

Item	Calories
1 serving *Fish and Vegetables à l'Orange*	188
1 medium baked potato with	145
2 tablespoons *Mollenized Sour Cream*	24
3 slices whole wheat bread with	183
3 tablespoons apple butter	111
2 cups strawberries, sliced	88
1 cup skim milk	88
	827

Total calories: 2,012

*Recipes for italicized dishes begin on page 237. Recipes are arranged according to alphabetical order for easy reference.

(Continued)

2,000-CALORIE PLAN – Continued
Week 1

Breakfast	Lunch	Dinner
WEDNESDAY		
1 cup apple juice 116	Spinach salad:	4 ounces cod, baked, broiled or poached 186
1 medium banana 101	2 cups shredded spinach 28	1 serving *Cheesy Potatoes* 190
1 cup Grape-Nuts with 404	½ cup sliced mushrooms 10	Relish plate:
1 cup skim milk 88	½ cup sliced beets 27	1 medium carrot, julienned 30
709	½ cup bean sprouts 23	½ cup broccoli flowerets 20
	½ cup zucchini strips 11	2 tablespoons *Buttermilk Dressing* 12
	2 tablespoons *Mustard Dressing* 18	2 slices whole wheat bread 122
	6 rye wafers 135	1 large apple 133
	1 large apple 133	1 cup skim milk 88
	1 cup pear nectar 125	**781**
	510	

Total calories: 2,000

Breakfast	Lunch	Dinner
THURSDAY		
1 cup orange juice 112	2 cups *Cucumber Soup* 110	2 *Vegetable Kabobs* 250
4 biscuits Shredded Wheat with 332	1 cup low-fat cottage cheese 164	1 serving *Rice Pilaf* 247
1 cup skim milk 88	2 slices pumpernickel bread 158	1 whole wheat roll 70
1 medium banana 101	1 large apple 133	1 medium navel orange 65
633	1 cup skim milk 88	1 cup skim milk 88
	653	**720**

Total calories: 2,006

FRIDAY

1 cup orange juice	112
3 servings *Cottage Cheese and Cinnamon Toast*	306
1 cup skim milk	88
	506

Mollen Milkshake	350
4 rye wafers	90
1 ounce part-skim mozzarella cheese	72
1 medium apple	87
1 medium navel orange	65
	664

2 cups cooked spaghetti with	384
1 cup tomato sauce and	70
½ cup cooked sliced mushrooms	10
Mixed salad:	
2 cups shredded lettuce	20
½ cup sliced radishes	10
½ cup sliced cucumbers	8
2 tablespoons *Italian Dressing*	5
2 slices whole wheat bread	122
1 medium apple	87
1 cup grapes	53
1 cup skim milk	88
	857

Total calories: 2,027

SATURDAY

1 cup orange juice	112
2 slices whole wheat toast with	122
2 tablespoons fruit preserves	108
1 cup oatmeal with	146
1 cup skim milk	88
1 medium apple	87
	663

Fruit salad:	
1 large apple, diced	133
1 medium navel orange, diced	65
1 medium banana, sliced	101
1 cup grapes	53
¼ cup *Fruit Salad Dressing*	32
6 slices melba toast	90
1 cup skim milk	88
	562

2 servings *Low-Fat Spinach Bake*	332
1 medium baked potato with	145
2 tablespoons *Mollenized Sour Cream*	24
2 whole wheat dinner rolls	140
2 cups strawberries, sliced	88
1 cup skim milk	88
	817

Total calories: 2,042

(Continued)

2,000-CALORIE PLAN – Continued
Week 2
10% Calories from Fat

Breakfast		Lunch		Dinner	
SUNDAY					
½ cup apple juice	58	1 cup chicken consommé	39	1 serving *Tart and Creamy Coleslaw*	24
½ medium cantaloupe	94	3 *Fruit Blintzes*	210	4 ounces pink salmon,* baked, broiled or poached	160
1 cup 40% Bran Flakes with	146	6 slices melba toast	90	1 cup steamed broccoli	40
1 cup skim milk	88	1 cup low-fat cottage cheese with	164	2 servings *Stuffed Potatoes*	140
2 slices whole wheat toast with	122	2 medium tomatoes, wedged	66	2 whole wheat dinner rolls with	140
2 tablespoons apple butter	74	1 cup skim milk	88	1 teaspoon margarine	34
		herbal tea with lemon wedge	5	1 large apple	133
				1 cup skim milk	88
	582		662		759

Total calories: 2,003

*Chinook and sockeye have a higher fat and calorie content.

Breakfast		Lunch		Dinner	
MONDAY					
1 cup orange juice	112	1 cup clear vegetable soup	64	1 serving *Cucumber-Onion Salad*	27
2 slices French toast made with	122	2 slices rye bread	122	1½ servings *Hearty Halibut*	225
2 slices whole wheat bread		2 ounces part-skim American cheese, sliced	180	1 small baked potato	90
1 egg	78	1 medium banana	101	2 medium carrots, sliced and steamed	60
1 tablespoon skim milk	5	1 large apple	133	2 slices whole wheat bread with	122
nonstick vegetable spray	0	1 cup skim milk	88	1 teaspoon margarine	34
Topped with				2 servings *Pears in Wine*	180
2 tablespoons fruit preserves	108			1 cup skim milk	88
1 cup skim milk	88				
	513		688		826

Total calories: 2,027

TUESDAY

Item	Calories
1 cup pineapple juice	140
1 cup Raisin Bran with	168
1 cup skim milk	88
2 slices whole wheat toast with	122
2 tablespoons apple butter	74
	592
Mollen Milkshake	350
6 rye wafers	135
2 ounces part-skim American cheese, sliced	180
1 large apple	133
	798
4 servings *Stuffed Celery*	52
1 serving *Poached Chicken Breast*	150
2 servings *Tangy Cauliflower*	54
2 slices whole wheat bread	122
1 cup juice-packed sliced peaches	58
1 medium navel orange	65
1 cup skim milk	88
	589

Total calories: 1,979

WEDNESDAY

Item	Calories
1 cup orange juice	112
½ medium cantaloupe	94
2 slices raisin toast with	140
1 teaspoon margarine and a	34
sprinkle of cinnamon	0
1 large apple	133
1 cup skim milk	88
	601
⅔ cup tomato juice	34
1 cup clear vegetable soup	64
2 ounces part-skim mozzarella cheese, cubed	144
6 rye wafers	135
1 large apple, wedged	133
1 cup skim milk	88
	598
2 servings *Triple Bean Salad*	122
1½ servings *Red Snapper*	170
1 medium baked potato with	145
2 tablespoons *Mollenized Sour Cream*	24
2 servings *Orangey Carrots*	74
2 slices whole wheat bread with	122
2 teaspoons fruit preserves	36
1 cup skim milk	88
	781

Total calories: 1,980

THURSDAY

Item	Calories
1 cup grapefruit juice	96
1 cup blueberries	82
1 cup 40% Bran Flakes with	146
1 cup skim milk	88
1 medium navel orange	65
	477
Relish plate:	
1 medium carrot, julienned	30
1 large stalk celery, julienned	9
2 tablespoons *Buttermilk Dressing*	12
6 large graham crackers with	330
2 tablespoons *Mollenized Sour Cream*	24
1 large pear	122
1 cup skim milk	88
	615
4 *Stuffed Mushrooms*	44
1 serving *Oriental Chicken*	205
1 cup cooked brown rice	232
½ cup low-fat cottage cheese	82
2 slices whole wheat bread with	122
1 teaspoon margarine	34
1 large apple	133
1 cup skim milk	88
	940

Total calories: 2,032

(Continued)

2,000-CALORIE PLAN – Continued
Week 2

Breakfast	Lunch	Dinner

FRIDAY

Breakfast		Lunch		Dinner	
¼ medium honeydew melon	116	Cottage cheese and fresh fruit plate:		4 ounces cod, baked, broiled or poached	186
3 servings *Cottage Cheese and Cinnamon Toast*	306	1 cup low-fat cottage cheese	164	1 cup steamed cauliflower	28
1 large apple	133	1 large apple, wedged	133	2 whole wheat dinner rolls with	140
1 cup skim milk	88	1 cup strawberries, sliced	44	1 teaspoon margarine	34
	643	4 medium prunes, sliced	82	2 servings *Fruit Ambrosia*	120
		1 medium navel orange, wedged	65	1 cup skim milk	88
		6 slices melba toast	90		596
		1 cup skim milk	88		
			666		

Total calories: 1,905

SATURDAY

Breakfast		Lunch		Dinner	
1 cup orange juice	112	Yogurt-pineapple refresher:		Tuna melt:	
2 slices whole wheat toast with	122	1 cup plain, low-fat yogurt, mixed with	144	Broil	
2 tablespoons apple butter	74	¾ cup crushed pineapple packed in its own juice and	113	2 slices lightly toasted whole wheat bread topped with	122
¾ cup Grape-Nuts with	303	2 tablespoons raisins	62	3 ounces water-packed tuna and	108
1 cup skim milk	88	1 slice rye bread	61	2 ounces part-skim American cheese, shredded	140
	699	8 rye wafers	180	1 large apple	133
		1 medium apple	87	1 12-ounce light beer	95
		1 cup skim milk	88		598
			735		

Week 3
15% Calories from Fat

Breakfast	Lunch	Dinner
SUNDAY		
1 cup orange juice 112	Tossed tuna salad:	2 servings *Marinated Vegetables* 46
1 medium banana 101	4 ounces water-packed tuna 144	1½ cups cooked spaghetti with 288
1 cup All-Bran with 214	1 cup shredded romaine	¾ cup tomato sauce 52
1 cup skim milk 88	lettuce 10	Dinner salad:
515	1 cup shredded red-leaf	2 cups shredded lettuce 20
	lettuce 10	½ cup croutons 28
	1 medium tomato, wedged 33	2 tablespoons *Italian Dressing* 5
	½ medium cucumber, sliced 15	1 slice whole wheat bread with 61
	2 ounces low-fat string	2 teaspoons margarine 68
	cheese, shredded 180	3 medium plums 108
	2 tablespoons *Mustard*	1 cup skim milk 88
	Dressing 18	764
	4 rye wafers 90	
	1 large apple 133	
	1 cup skim milk 88	
	721	

Total calories: 2,000

(Continued)

2,000-CALORIE PLAN–Continued
Week 3

Breakfast		Lunch		Dinner	

MONDAY

Breakfast		Lunch		Dinner	
1 cup apple juice	116	Cheese crisps:		1½ servings *Marinated Halibut*	216
1 cup oatmeal with	146	Broil		2 servings *Asparagus Delight*	32
2 tablespoons raisins and	62	2 12-inch tortillas sprinkled	252	2 servings *Parslied Potatoes*	132
1 cup skim milk	88	with		2 slices whole wheat bread with	122
1 *Mollen Muffin*	103	2 ounces part-skim American	180	2 teaspoons margarine	68
	515	cheese, shredded, and		1 large apple	133
		½ medium tomato, chopped	17	1 cup skim milk	88
		1 *Banana Pop*	60		791
		1 medium navel orange	65		
		1 cup skim milk	88		
			662		

Total calories: 1,968

TUESDAY

Breakfast		Lunch		Dinner	
1 cup apple juice	116	Cucumber boat:		3 *Chicken Kabobs*	102
2 whole wheat English muffins with	280	1 medium cucumber stuffed	30	1 serving *Spinach Casserole*	203
1 tablespoon peanut butter and	95	with		1 medium baked potato with	145
1 tablespoon honey	64	3 ounces water-packed tuna	108	2 tablespoons *Mollenized*	
1 large apple	133	2 slices whole wheat bread with	122	*Sour Cream*	24
1 cup skim milk	88	2 teaspoons margarine	68	1 medium navel orange	65
	776	2 medium plums	72	1 cup skim milk	88
		1 medium banana	101		627
		1 cup *Sparkling Juice* (grape)	84		
			585		

Total calories: 1,988

WEDNESDAY

	Calories
1 cup mixed juice:	
½ cup pineapple juice mixed with	70
½ cup grapefruit juice	48
4 biscuits Shredded Wheat with	332
1½ cups skim milk	132
1 slice whole wheat toast with	61
1 teaspoon margarine	34
	677

	Calories
1½ servings Turkey Chili	233
Tossed salad:	
1 cup shredded romaine lettuce	10
1 cup shredded red-leaf lettuce	10
1 medium tomato, sliced	32
⅛ avocado, sliced	45
2 tablespoons Italian Dressing	5
1 slice whole wheat bread	61
1 large apple	133
1 cup skim milk	88
	617

	Calories
1½ servings Sole with Yogurt Sauce	186
2 servings Mashed Squash	122
1 serving Ambrosia Medley	95
1 whole wheat dinner roll with	70
1 teaspoon margarine	34
1 large apple	133
1 cup skim milk	88
	728

Total calories: 2,022

THURSDAY

	Calories
¾ cup peach nectar	101
½ cup All-Bran with	107
2 tablespoons raisins and	62
1 cup skim milk	88
1 slice whole wheat toast with	61
1 teaspoon margarine	34
1 medium apple	87
	540

	Calories
Fruit salad:	
1 large apple, sliced	133
1 medium navel orange, sliced	65
½ cup grapes	53
1 medium banana, sliced	101
½ cup Fruit Salad Dressing	64
6 slices melba toast	90
2 ounces part-skim American cheese, cubed	180
½ cup skim milk	44
	730

	Calories
⅔ cup vegetable juice	34
1½ servings Sole and Broccoli with Rice	402
2 slices whole wheat bread with	122
1 teaspoon margarine	34
1 cup strawberries, sliced	44
1 cup skim milk	88
	724

Total calories: 1,994

(Continued)

2,000-CALORIE PLAN – Continued
Week 3

Breakfast		Lunch		Dinner	
FRIDAY					
¾ cup prune juice	138	Peanut butter and banana sandwich:		*Mollen Milkshake*	350
2 *Mollen Muffins* with	206	2 slices whole wheat bread	122	Turkey sandwich:	
1 tablespoon honey	64	2 teaspoons peanut butter	64	2 slices rye bread	122
1 cup strawberries, sliced	44	1 small banana, sliced	85	1 tablespoon low-fat mayonnaise	35
1 cup skim milk	88	1 cup grapes	53	3 ounces cold turkey breast, sliced	115
	540	1 large apple	133	2 ounces part-skim mozzarella cheese, sliced	144
		1 cup skim milk	88	1 medium navel orange	65
			545		831
Total calories: 1,916					
SATURDAY					
1 cup orange juice	112	Health salad:		⅔ cup tomato juice	34
1 cup Grape-Nuts with	404	2 cups shredded lettuce	20	1 serving *Poached Chicken Breast*	150
1 medium banana, sliced, and	101	1 cup sliced cucumbers	16	¾ cup steamed green beans with	25
1½ cups skim milk	132	1 medium tomato, sliced	32	½ cup cooked sliced mushrooms	10
	749	1 tablespoon sunflower seeds	45	1 cup mashed potatoes with	140
		2 ounces low-fat string cheese, shredded	180	2 teaspoons margarine	68
		2 tablespoons *Buttermilk Dressing*	12	1 large apple	133
		4 rye wafers	90	1 12-ounce light beer	95
		1 medium apple	87		655
		1 cup skim milk	88		
			570		
Total calories: 1,974					

Week 4
20% Calories from Fat

Breakfast		Lunch		Dinner	
SUNDAY					
1 cup orange juice	112	1 serving *Lean Lasagna*	275	1½ servings *Patio Potato Salad*	155
2 servings *Whole Wheat Bran Pancakes* with	276	Tossed salad:		4 *Chicken Kabobs*	136
1 tablespoon peanut butter and	95	2 cups shredded lettuce	20	2 whole wheat dinner rolls with	140
2 tablespoons apple butter	74	1 medium tomato, wedged	32	2 teaspoons margarine	68
1 cup skim milk	88	2 tablespoons *Italian Dressing*	5	3 medium plums	108
	645	1 serving *Art's Brown Apple*	140	1 medium apple	87
		1 cup skim milk	88	1 cup *Spicy Lemon Iced Tea*	64
			560		758
Total calories: 1,963					
MONDAY					
1 cup grapefruit juice	96	2 servings *Stuffed Tomato Salad*	256	3 servings *Orange-Carrot Salad*	147
4 biscuits Shredded Wheat with	332	1 ounce part-skim American cheese, sliced	90	1½ servings *Sole Florentine*	195
1 medium banana, sliced, and	101	6 rye wafers	135	1 medium baked potato with	145
1½ cups skim milk	132	1 large apple	133	2 tablespoons *Mollenized Sour Cream*	24
	661	1 cup skim milk	88	1 medium navel orange	65
			702	1 cup skim milk	88
					664
Total calories: 2,027					

(Continued)

2,000-CALORIE PLAN – *Continued*
Week 4

	Breakfast	Lunch	Dinner
TUESDAY			
	1 cup grapefruit juice — 96	⅔ cup tomato juice — 34	1 serving *Waldorf Salad* — 110
	1 cup strawberries, sliced — 44	1 serving *Tangy Chicken Salad* — 230	1 serving *Fish Creole* — 238
	2 slices whole wheat toast with — 122	on a bed of lettuce — 15	1 cup steamed brussels sprouts — 56
	2 teaspoons margarine and — 68	6 slices melba toast — 90	2 slices pumpernickel bread with — 158
	2 tablespoons fruit preserves — 108	2 *Pineapple Pops* — 180	1 teaspoon margarine — 34
	1 cup skim milk — 88	1 cup skim milk — 88	1 large apple — 133
			1 cup skim milk — 88
	526	637	817

Total calories: 1,980

	Breakfast	Lunch	Dinner
WEDNESDAY			
	1 papaya — 116	2 cups *Cucumber Soup* — 110	4 ounces baked turkey breast fillets — 153
	1 whole wheat English muffin with — 140	2 slices whole wheat bread with — 122	2 servings *Spinach Royale* — 60
	1 tablespoon peanut butter — 95	2 teaspoons margarine — 68	1 medium baked potato with — 145
	1 cup oatmeal with — 146	1 large apple — 133	2 tablespoons *Mollenized Sour Cream* — 24
	2 tablespoons raisins and — 62	1 cup skim milk — 88	1 whole wheat dinner roll with — 70
	1 cup skim milk — 88		1 teaspoon margarine — 34
	1 medium apple — 87		1 medium banana — 101
			1 cup skim milk — 88
	734	521	675

Total calories: 1,930

THURSDAY

1 cup apricot nectar	142
2 servings *Whole Wheat Bran Pancakes* with	276
2 tablespoons fruit preserves	108
1 large apple	133
1 cup skim milk	88

1 *Chicken Pocket Sandwich*	284
3 cups plain popcorn (air popped)	70
1 medium banana	101
1 cup skim milk	88
	543

1 *Chilled Shrimp and Mushroom Kabob*	200
½ cup cooked brown rice	116
½ cup peas	57
1 serving *Pineapple Baked Apple*	160
1 slice whole wheat bread with	61
1 teaspoon margarine	34
1 cup skim milk	88
	716

Total calories: 2,006

FRIDAY

½ medium grapefruit	41
2 slices whole wheat toast with	122
2 teaspoons peanut butter	64
½ cup Grape-Nuts with	202
1 cup skim milk	88

1 serving *Turkey-Squash Bake*	230
1 cup low-fat cottage cheese	164
4 rye wafers	90
1 large apple	133
1 serving *Fruit Slush*	60
1 cup skim milk	88
	517

Dr. Art's Avocado Omelet	157
2 whole wheat English muffins with	280
2 teaspoons margarine	68
2 cups diced fresh pineapple	138
1 cup skim milk	88
	731

Total calories: 2,013

SATURDAY

1 cup pear nectar	125
2 *Mollen Muffins* with	206
1 tablespoon honey	64
1 large apple	133
1 cup skim milk	88

1 serving *Fish and Vegetables à l'Orange*	188
2 medium ears corn on the cob with	140
2 teaspoons margarine	68
½ cup peas	57
1 slice pumpernickel bread	79
1 cup juice-packed fruit cocktail	74
1 cup skim milk	88
	616

1½ servings *Saucy Chicken and Cheese*	285
1 cup steamed eggplant	38
1 cup steamed broccoli	40
2 slices whole wheat bread with	122
2 teaspoons margarine	68
1 12-ounce light beer	95
	648

Total calories: 1,958

"The best reward was my parents' reaction when I went home to Philadelphia to visit them," says Jay. "They didn't even recognize me when I got off the plane. They were so pleased! It really gave me the incentive to keep it up. Now I'm addicted to this new eating style. I love all the grains and fruits. I can't believe the way I used to eat. No wonder I felt so lousy. I thought that was just me, just the way I am. Not so. I love my new energy."

A Matter of Lifestyle

The stories are endless. You'll hear many more before you finish reading this book. Some day you, too, can tell your own story about your body makeover. To make your wish come true—to make the Mollen Method work for you permanently—is to make it your new lifestyle.

Dieting for four weeks and going back to your old style of living isn't going to work. Exercising one day here and one day there isn't going to work either. It takes a new commitment, as I told you in Chapter 1; a good attitude, as I emphasized in Chapter 2; a will to be healthy, as I pointed out in Chapter 3; and an exercise plan that will become a part of your life, as I explained in Chapter 4.

Now you've learned all about eating properly. As long as you stick with it I can guarantee you'll lose weight and gain health and energy.

So, do as I once did and take it one day at a time. Each day you'll feel a little stronger, a little healthier, a little slimmer and a little more pleased with yourself. What more could you ask for?

Chapter 6

S-T-R-E-T-C-H !

Stretch thy muscles and joints so thy aching bones will be relieved and thou shall feel good again.
— Anonymous

The Eastern civilizations believe that the key to longevity is a supple spine. Mobility in the joints, they say, will promote activity. An increase in activity means a more conditioned cardiovascular system and more alert mind, leading to a long life.

Stretching → Mobile joints → Activity →
Cardiovascular fitness → Alert mind → Longevity

So stretching is an important part of staying fit. For instance, students of Hatha Yoga who do lots of stretching become extremely flexible as they enhance the elasticity of their muscles. However, stretching will not promote weight loss, nor will it build a strong heart. It is not considered aerobic exercise, and therefore, cannot take the place of your ten minutes a day. In fact, you shouldn't even think of stretching as exercise. Rather, consider it something you should do to make your exercise easier. So when I recommend stretching before aerobics, don't think that I've tricked you into doing more exercise than the minimal daily dose. I'm simply suggesting that stretching will make you feel better.

Just look at cats. They aren't exactly known as energetic creatures. All they do is sleep and eat, rarely engaging in anything more strenuous than play. But before they even *move*, they take a long stretch. That's because it makes them feel good. It'll make you feel good, too.

201

Why Stretching Is Important

Many people plunge into an exercise program without stretching, or warming up, the muscles that they've allowed to become soft and weak. They simply start jogging, bicycling or jumping rope and try to regain the timing they had so long ago without preparing their muscles for this new demand. As a result, they experience an injury of some sort: torn muscles, sprains or even worse. The injury stops the exercise program temporarily, at best, or stops it totally.

Stretching is especially important for the overweight because their extra pounds put more stress on their joints and muscles. Those areas can therefore be injured quite easily. But whether you're overweight or slim, stretching is a must. Ninety-five percent of the athletic injuries I treat in my office could have been prevented by simply stretching before exercise.

One of the classic excuses people use to avoid following the Mollen Method is, "I've developed an injury, I *can't* exercise." As a result, they slide back into the vicious cycle of overeating, inactivity, weight gain and fad dieting. If all of this sounds familiar, don't feel bad. The first thing you must do is learn to stretch and take it seriously. Then you'll greatly reduce your chances of getting injured and excuses will be harder to find.

Stretching is a natural thing to do. Consider how often you get out of bed in the morning or out of an armchair after a lazy night of watching television, and lift your arms way over your head and stretch for the ceiling. Feels good, doesn't it?

Well, that's what I'm going to have you do each day before you exercise. That's right, just stretch. Go ahead . . . lean back, reach those arms high and stretch. It's not hard; it doesn't take much time; and it makes you feel better.

Not only will stretching help you prevent injuries, but it will lessen the aches and pains of your exercise regimen. And if you do get an injury, it will help you heal more quickly.

Now that's not a bad payoff for something that comes naturally, feels good and doesn't require a lot of effort!

Paying the Penalty

What happens if you *don't* stretch? I'll let one of my patients tell you:

"I started playing racquetball several years ago and loved the game from the start," says Bob. "Not only was it fun, but once I found myself a regular partner who would play every morning before work, I really started to lose weight.

"Racquetball did the trick—when I could play. But I couldn't *always* play. It seemed that either my partner was injured or I was. Racquetball's a pretty demanding sport and one of us was always pulling a muscle or straining something in our shoulders, back, legs or arms. If one was hurt the other didn't play—and didn't get any exercise. I remember one occasion when I pulled a muscle in my thigh and couldn't play for three weeks. Naturally, I gained weight during that time.

"So I started stretching before playing and the injuries stopped. I convinced my partner to stretch too, and now we do it together every day. It's made a world of difference, not only in the amount of injuries we have, but in the game as well. Now, when an injury does occur, the recovery time is shorter.

"In fact, we've both gotten better at the game. This is due mostly to practice, but I think it's partly due to an increase in flexibility. Now when I move to pick up a shot, I'm able to stretch farther and keep my balance."

That's a good example of why you should stretch before exercising. Until Bob learned the importance of stretching he had problems sustaining an exercise program. But unlike many people, he stuck it out and kept going back to his exercise program until he learned how to do it right. He learned how to stretch.

A Little Magic

As you can see, a few minutes of stretching will make a big difference in the way you play your game, in the way you feel, even in the way you look!

You might be wondering what stretching does for your body that's so important. After all, when you were a kid and played football or baseball you didn't stretch that much, and you don't remember hurting yourself or having sore muscles.

Well, we've learned a lot since then. Back in those days, coaches were just as anxious as you to get you onto the playing field, diamond or court and begin the game. They didn't understand the value of stretching. They do now. I doubt there's a high school coach anywhere who doesn't make his team warm up before they practice.

The real reason you were able to escape injury back then is that you had age on your side. But now you don't. You were more supple then, so your risk of getting an injury was much lower.

Stretching before exercising is important primarily because it helps to get blood flowing to the muscles. As you warm up, your body diverts blood flow to your muscles from your internal organs in order to prepare them for exercise. This is how stretching prevents injury.

For the same reason, stretching is also important after exercise. (This is known as the cool-down.) During exercise, your heart is pumping efficiently and the blood is flowing to the muscles. Then suddenly you stop exercising. Cooling down allows time for your muscles to transfer the blood back to other areas. Stretching, walking or a combination of the two are good ways to cool down.

A sudden stop after hard exercise sends messages to the brain suggesting that the elevation of blood pressure and heart rate must be maintained. These messages cause a release of catecholamines (nervous system stimulants) which attempt to maintain the elevated blood pressure and pulse rate. The result can be an overstimulation of the heart, causing an irregular heartbeat and even cardiac arrest. So I cannot overemphasize the importance of warming up before *and* cooling down after exercise. It's simply a good exercise habit.

Of course, not *everyone* has to stretch in order to avoid injuries. Some people—but very few—are just naturally more flexible and their muscles are more elastic than others. They can bend where others buckle. However, as we age we lose a tremendous amount of flexibility and elasticity in our muscles. So for the majority of us, it is very important to stretch to avoid injuries. It is doubly important to do so at the start of an exercise program when everything is new to you and your body is the most vulnerable. In order to succeed on my program, you must exercise every day. And it won't be much fun if your calves, hips or back are aching.

Flexibility Versus Joint Movement

So an important step in gaining control of your health is daily stretching. When people talk about stretching, they're referring to flexibility. Flexibility is defined as the ability to move a joint through a range of motion, whether it's a hip joint, knee joint, elbow joint or foot joint. The greater the range of motion, the greater the flexibility.

Joint looseness, on the other hand, is different from flexibility. Increased joint movement is simply greater flexion or extension of the joint itself and does not necessarily involve the muscle groups of the joint.

Bob's problems on the racquetball court occurred because his muscles weren't flexible enough for the demands of the sport. They were too "tight," too inflexible. The injuries came from pulling the muscles near the joints, tendons and ligaments past the point where they could stretch easily. He tore the muscles and strained them. That's what aches and pains, even little ones, are—slight pulls and tears. The worse the pull or tear, the greater the pain.

The little aches and pains you may experience are not uncommon. After all, there are many different muscles in the human body and some of them will ache from time to time no matter how well conditioned you are (or aren't) and no matter how flexible you are (or aren't).

The body has numerous muscles and each sport that you participate in can affect them differently. So for each sport there may be different muscles and joints that need different types of stretching exercises. Different exercises also may produce different aches and pains. For instance, a runner in excellent shape who goes skiing for the first time without stretching is liable to discover muscles he or she never knew existed.

Once you've picked the exercise or exercises you're going to follow, stretch the appropriate muscles and prepare them for the workout. It'll prevent you from using the universal excuse: "I hurt too much."

As for the amount of time you spend stretching, I recommend *at least* five minutes. You should stretch after exercise, too. Remember, just because you have some aches and pains after exercising doesn't mean you're injured. It just means you've exercised. A little stretching immediately afterwards and even again the next day, if necessary, can help to reduce these aches and pains. Walking after exercise, in my mind, is a great way to stretch. After running a marathon, I ache all over. So I stretch and walk a lot. And the best thing for me to do the next day is to walk a few miles to stretch out my sore muscles.

How to Stretch

There are basically three ways to stretch muscles. The first is ballistic-type stretching which involves bouncing up and down, like jumping jacks. Because of its jerky and jarring movements, this type of stretching can actually cause injuries and muscle soreness. I'd suggest that you avoid it.

A second type of stretching is a passive type of stretching exercise which requires some kind of resistance. An example would be reaching down to touch your toes and then grabbing hold of your toes and pulling yourself all the way down. This type of stretching can also cause an injury if you force a muscle and joint to move farther than normal. It is sometimes done with the help of a partner, who may unintentionally force an injury by pushing or pulling too hard. For example, someone pulling your arms together behind you as you attempt to clasp your hands behind your back could result in tendonitis in the shoulder. This type of stretching is best left to the more experienced or flexible athlete. If you do choose to do it, however, I'd suggest avoiding a partner.

The best type of stretching is "passive" or "static" stretching. In this method a particular position is gently held for a 30-second period, released

THE FLEXIBILITY TEST

How flexible are you? Let's find out.

Hip flexion is considered to be the most important measurement of flexibility because it involves movement of the hips, hamstrings and calves. This simple test will give you an idea of how flexible you are. Sit on the floor with your legs together and place a yardstick by your side with the 10-inch mark at your ankle bone. High numbers should be facing out. Stretch forward (but do not strain!) and, using your fingertips as the gauge, measure how far forward you can stretch. The following will give you an indication as to how you measure up in the flexibility area:

Males	Rating	Females
10-11 inches	Poor	10-11 inches
12-13 inches	Fair	12-13 inches
14-18 inches	Average	14-21 inches
19-21 inches	Good	22-24 inches
22-23 inches	Excellent	25-28 inches

Females generally have greater elasticity than men and will be able to stretch slightly farther.

Sports that require more flexibility than others are swimming, running and fencing. Greater flexibility will improve performance in these sports.

and then repeated three times. This type of stretching is the safest, and if done properly—that is, without pushing or pulling beyond what is naturally comfortable—it will enhance flexibility the most. There is generally less muscle soreness with this type of stretching. It's the same technique often used in Hatha Yoga. I recommend it highly for the beginning exercise enthusiast or "not-so-enthusiast."

Getting Down to Specifics

Who can benefit from stretching? Everyone. That's right, no exceptions. However, certain sports make greater demands on certain parts of your body, and these require additional stretching. I recommend a good all-body stretch every day, but if you're pushed for time—honestly pushed for time and not just being lazy—then stretch only the muscles you're going to use.

Here are some common forms of exercises and the muscle groups that must be stretched before beginning each. You can consult the exercise routines that follow for specific instructions.

Running: Stretch the quadriceps muscles, hamstring muscles, groin muscles, knee joints, calf muscles and Achilles' tendons.

Bicycling: Stretch the quadriceps muscles, knee joints, inguinal muscles (pubic muscles) and lower back.

Swimming: Stretch mostly the leg muscles, calves, hamstrings, Achilles' tendons, and upper-body and shoulder muscles.

Aerobic Dancing: Stretch all upper-body and lower-body muscles. A good aerobics class will incorporate at least five minutes of stretching in the routine.

Skiing: Stretch the quadriceps muscles, hips, knees, calves and Achilles' tendons. In addition, emphasis should be placed on stretching the lower back muscles.

Racquet Sports (tennis and racquetball): Stretch the knees, calves, quadriceps muscles, hamstrings and especially for women, the Achilles' tendons. (Women's Achilles' tendons are often shorter than men's because of the wearing of high-heeled shoes.) Upper-body stretches for the shoulder and elbow also must be done to avoid tennis elbow.

Weight Training: For weight training, the total body stretch is important. Because weight training may often cause elbow, shoulder or neck pain, it's also important to emphasize upper-body stretching exercises. And as training increases the size of your muscles (this is called hypertrophy), the flexibility of the muscles will decrease unless you routinely stretch. In fact, the Herculean-type (muscle-bound) build requires stretching exercise to prevent loss of muscle flexibility.

YOUR DAILY STRETCHES

Stretches should be held in a stationary position for a minimum of 30 seconds. They should be repeated at least three times if not otherwise specified. It is important not to bounce or strain when stretching as this may cause a slight tearing of muscles.

Lower Back and Back of Legs (Hamstrings)

Place your feet together and bend at the waist, allowing your arms to hang down as far as possible. Return to the starting position. Raise your arms above your head and stand on tiptoes. Hold.

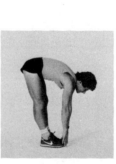
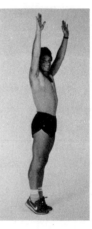

Groin and Buttocks (Inguinals)

Sit on the floor with your knees bent and the soles of your feet together. Push your knees down to the floor as far as possible. Hold.

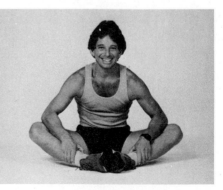

Lower Back, Entire Spine

Sit with your knees bent and soles together. Take hold of your toes and pull your body forward, getting your head as close to your toes as you can. Keep your knees as flat as possible while bending down. Hold.

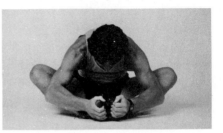

Back of Legs (Hamstrings)

Lean against a wall with outstretched arms. Bend the knee of your right leg and place the left leg straight out behind it, with the heel of your foot on the floor. Hold. Switch legs and repeat.

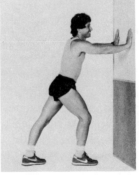

Quadriceps and Knees

Stand erect. Grab your right foot with your right hand, bending your knee toward your back. Hold. Repeat with the left leg. You can use your free hand for support if necessary.

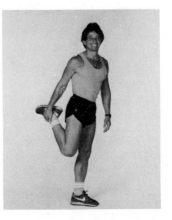

(Continued)

YOUR DAILY STRETCHES—Continued

Achilles' Tendons, Calves and Feet

Stand on a step and hang your heel over the step, one foot at a time. Alternate and repeat 30 times.

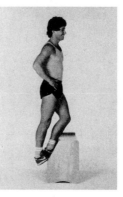

Waist

Stand erect. Lean to the right, raising your left arm and moving your right down, close to your right leg. Do not move your hips. Hold. Repeat with the left side. Repeat 20 times.

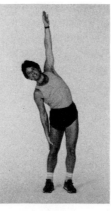

Abdomen

Lie on the floor and bend your knees to protect your lower back. Place your arms across your chest and gently raise your torso. Repeat 20 times.

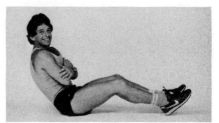

Shoulders and Upper Back

Stand erect. Lean forward and stretch your arms straight back, clasping your hands. Reach as high as possible. Hold.

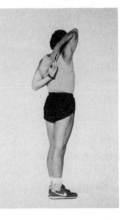

Shoulders and Elbows

Stand erect. Place your left arm behind your back and your right arm over your right shoulder. Attempt to clasp your hands behind you. Use a towel to join hands if you're unable to do this. Hold.

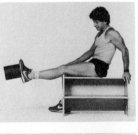

Knees

Sit on a table with your knee on the edge and a 10- to 15-pound weight on your foot or ankle. (A paint can filled partially with sand works nicely.) Lift your leg straight out and then bend it to an angle of 30 to 45 degrees. Repeat 20 times. Switch the weight to the other foot and repeat.

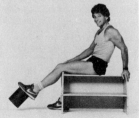

(Continued)

Shins

Sit on a table with your ankle on the edge and a 5- to 10-pound weight on your foot or ankle. (Again a paint can filled with sand will work nicely.) Bend your ankle upward, flexing it back and forth. Repeat 20 times. Switch the weight to the other foot and repeat. This exercise will help prevent shin splints.

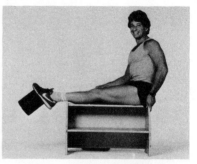

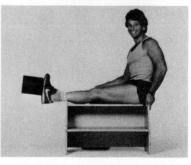

Lower Back

Get down on the floor and support yourself with your toes and the palms of your hands. Arch your lower back and lift your head up. Hold your stomach and buttocks tight. Hold for five seconds. Relax and repeat.

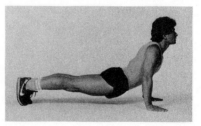

Chapter 7

THE BUSY LIFE OF THE BUSINESS EXECUTIVE

It's not easy climbing the ladder to success, especially if you're out of shape. Staying *in* shape, though, can be hard to manage when you must deal with the business (and social) pressures that go with the job—like business lunches, cocktail parties, conferences and travel (which means meals) away from home. Exercise and diet become crucial!

Early in their careers successful business men and women are quick to realize that appearance is important. Just as they must have control over the company's cash flow or inventory, they know they also must have control over their personal inventory. After all, they represent their company, and they understand that the clients or customers they meet see *them* as the company, whether it's a corporation or a small private business. This is why so many men and women in the business world end up in my office looking for diet and fitness advice.

Executive Excuses

Needless to say, I've heard *all* the excuses. Here's one I hear time and again: "Look, Doc, I really blew it last night. I had a huge steak, baked potato with sour cream and butter, drinks before dinner, wine with dinner, after-dinner drinks and even dessert."

I ask why.

"Well, I got a promotion and the boss insisted on taking me out to dinner. How could I refuse?"

Naturally, that doesn't happen all the time, but it happens more often than it should (I'm referring to the gluttony, not the promotion). Or perhaps you can relate to this one:

"He was an important client and I was sure I had the sale when he said he was hungry. So what could I do? I took him to dinner, of course. You don't want to know what we had . . . but I made the sale, isn't that what counts?"

Or how about this one:

"Well, I can't help it. I mean, the boss took me to lunch three times this last week. Can you believe it? Three times! That's how pleased he is with me lately. So, naturally, I didn't stay on the diet. What was I supposed to say, 'No, thanks, I'd rather stay in the office and eat carrot sticks'?"

I think bosses or chief executive officers (CEOs as they are referred to in the corporate structure) should reward employees with money for lost weight and exercise equipment for big sales instead of food and drinks. In fact, I know of a few CEOs who could use this incentive program themselves.

In all fairness, though, the corporate world is starting to take notice of the benefits of a healthy lifestyle to their employees. Some companies have instituted smoking bans and many offer stop-smoking, weight loss and fitness programs for employees. Some are even offering rewards in money and time off for attaining short-range health-oriented goals. In fact, corporations such as Greyhound, Continental Homes, Bonne Belle, and Talley Industries have developed programs which offer employees incentives for improving their health and fitness. Corporations are realizing that these personal accomplishments among their employees are resulting in increased productivity and creativity at work.

The old stereotype of a top corporate executive was a paunchy, out-of-shape-looking guy with a cigar hanging out of his mouth. Not so anymore. In fact, more and more CEOs are in *better* shape than the average person. They realize the importance of representing their company in the best possible way, which includes the establishment of leadership and direction—not simply in financial profits, but in health as well.

For instance, John Teets, the CEO and chairman of the board of the Greyhound Corporation with over 30,000 employees, has recognized the importance of exercise and diet for the last 20 years. He exercises an hour every day.

And then there's Bill Mallender, the CEO of Talley Industries, who has 14 subsidiary companies to control. A few years ago he found himself getting slightly out of control. He was 25 pounds overweight, did little exercise and was about to reach his 50th birthday. He knew changes had to be made so he began following my low-fat guidelines and started walking three miles daily. No doubt his productivity will soar—both financially and personally.

Or how about Lee Iacocca, chairman of the board of Chrysler Corporation. He exercises for 45 minutes every day and, on the weekend, "crews" for a half hour a day on a rowing machine.

Top executives like Iacocca, Teets and Mallender realize the importance of maintaining their health and fitness and you should also. If they can make time to exercise, so can you.

Don't Call "Time" for Travel

When it comes to finding an excuse not to exercise and eat healthfully, business travel takes the cake (yes, the pun is intended). The story usually goes like this:

"Last week was a total loss. I mean, I was traveling all week long. Five days out, five different cities and three different time zones. What could I do? If I didn't have jet lag then I had to be with a client early in the morning for a meeting and didn't have time to exercise. As for the diet, well, you know what airline food is like. And the restaurants in these cities are great and I was on an expense account! I'll start over again this week, I promise."

That's a promise too easily—and almost always—broken as soon as the next business trip comes around. I think the person who hasn't made that commitment to exercise when traveling and says, "I'm taking a trip; I'll continue my program when I come back," is on the wrong track. It's too easy to put it off and start the program again—some other day. With that attitude, tomorrow may never arrive. To me, this is not the image of a man or woman in control. And executives—successful executives—*are* in control. That's control not only of their business or company or corporation, but *self*-control.

If you don't believe me, go to any large office building or bank in your town during the lunch hour and find a place to simply sit and watch the people as they leave their offices. The successful people aren't difficult to spot. Some will be younger, some older; some dressed in suits, some wearing more casual clothing; some will have longer hair, some will have shorter hair. But you will soon realize that with very few exceptions they all have one thing in common.

Most of them are in shape.

There's no reason you can't be, either. The beauty of the Mollen Method is that it works at all times—anywhere. I know. I travel extensively. I sweep through city after city on the banquet circuit, talking to people and selling them on health. I understand how easy it is to use that hectic travel schedule as a handy excuse not to exercise or follow the diet. But look at my photo on the front of this book. Do I look out of shape? Do I look like I'm not in control of my diet? Of course not! No matter where I go I manage to work in an exercise routine.

I flew out of Phoenix not long ago just 30 minutes after giving a lecture and forgot my running shoes. I didn't realize it until the next morning. Did I skip exercise? No. I jogged in place in my stocking feet for 15 minutes and then did sit-ups and push-ups. My body felt better, more alert. But in my mind, I felt guilty. I was to lecture to 1,500 people about exercise, and because I forgot my shoes, I hadn't done much exercise that day. I was fortunate I wasn't asked to lead a run in the morning! They would have thought *I* was making an excuse . . . and you know how I admonish excuses.

But as you can see, all the "excuses" you can think of for not following my program are not valid excuses at all. That's because the Mollen Method is so easy to follow. Exercise? You can exercise anywhere. Diet? That's easy, too, because the program does not require any special foods. There are no weird concoctions or foods you can only find in a health food store. It's not the kind of diet that you can't follow if you left your powdered formula at home.

Hotel Room Exercise

I'm often the after-lunch or after-dinner speaker at banquets. I usually start my lectures on the importance of exercise, fat restriction and calorie control as the guests are taking their last bites of dessert. (I do this to motivate, not depress them.) At one lecture an executive interrupted to say that he exercised regularly by riding a bicycle, but since it's impossible to take his bicycle on trips with him he gets no exercise while away from home. I told him that was a poor excuse. I said he could simply do something else.

I suggested he put a jump rope in his briefcase and keep it there. Five to eight minutes a day of jumping rope in a hotel room is great exercise (see chart on pages 81-87). Or I suggested he try the "toilet seat step test." By stepping up and down on the toilet seat (providing the toilet seat is not a plastic one) in your hotel room for eight minutes, you will get an aerobic workout. (It's best to alternate feet while stepping up and down.) Or he could simply jog in place.

I have patients come into my office and say, "I was in New Orleans last week and stuck to the diet but I didn't exercise because we were staying at a hotel that didn't have a gym."

Again, no excuse. You can exercise wherever you go. Any city. Any hotel.

You can always exercise outside if you can't exercise inside. That includes just taking a walk. If it's $-34°F$ outside and you're a warm-weather bug like myself, then exercise inside. You can jump rope, run in place or do the "toilet seat step test."

But the problems of business travel don't start in the hotel room; they start as soon as you board the plane. So let's look at the traveling phase of your trip.

The Plane Facts

These days we travel at full throttle, taking quantum leaps from one coast to the other. On these journeys we're tempted with more drinks, meals and snacks than we really need.

So that's the first hurdle—taking charge of your eating habits, especially on the airplane where you probably eat because you're bored and not because you're hungry.

The first thing you can do when you know you're going to fly is call ahead to the airline and order a vegetarian meal or a fish meal, if you prefer. Most airlines will accommodate such requests. In fact, you'll most likely find this meal planning to your liking. The food actually tastes better, because special meals must be made fresh.

On shorter flights, you have snacks to deal with. What you get depends on the duration of the flight and time of day. It could be a small sandwich or simply a bag of nuts or chips.

Well, why bother snacking? Would you be snacking at this time of day if you were at home or in the office? Simply say "No, thank you." Just because it's free doesn't mean you have to eat it. Just think of all the calories you eat because something's "free" or "there." Remember, it's about 100 calories per bag for those nuts!

If you think you're going to need a snack, put an apple, orange or banana into your briefcase or purse and eat that. You'll not only save in calories but also eat higher quality food that is better for you.

We're not done with the flight yet. Drinks are served, remember?

One of the problems of drinking in flight is that alcohol is absorbed into your system at a faster rate when you're not moving around—and there's not much movement in the close quarters of an airline seat. One drink in the air is the equivalent of two on the ground, so minimize the amount of alcohol you consume when you're flying. Or have none. You can always have a club soda, orange juice or tomato juice. The juice is more nutritious, and of course, lower in calories than the alcohol.

If you're on the road and driving from city to city, following a good diet and exercise plan is a lot easier. Take fruit along with you. Bring a basket of nutritious, nonperishable foods that you enjoy so that you can pick and choose where and when to stop and eat. When you do stop at a restaurant, order light—fish, vegetable dishes, salads and the like. Most restaurants have all three, and more and more restaurants are featuring a salad bar.

What if they don't have salads, fish or vegetarian plates? There is still a solution. The restaurant is going to have baked potatoes and choices of vegetables served on the side. Just ask for two or three orders or however many orders it takes to fill you.

I've done just that. I've gone to restaurants and asked for two orders of carrots, two orders of baked potatoes, two orders of broccoli. That's my dinner. I'm usually asked, "Are you crazy?"

"Yes, crazy, but healthy," I tell them.

It is also important not to feel intimidated by another's eating habits. Eat whatever makes *you* feel good and helps keep you from gaining weight.

Coping with Jet Lag

Worse than the plane trip is the jet lag that too often follows it.

Most travelers have experienced jet lag in varying degrees at one time or another. It's that feeling of being out of sync with the world, being hours ahead of local time or hours behind. You end up sitting there bleary-eyed and sleepy when everyone else is fresh and wondering why you want to go to bed when the night is still young. Or eating breakfast when you feel like you haven't been to bed yet. Being out of sync means being out of sorts. And being out of sorts makes any eating program difficult—especially a diet plan. But, again, I have a solution.

Say you've gone from Los Angeles to New York and lost three hours of sleep. You've got to get up and start your working day when your body clock says it's the middle of the night. You feel worn out and the day is just starting. What do you do?

One of the best things to combat jet lag is exercise. I can guarantee that if you put in a minimum of ten minutes of exercise you'll feel better. It will make a significant difference in how you feel the rest of the day. You will find the following day that you're feeling even better and you're ready to resume your regular exercise program and normal eating schedule.

I understand that when you're tired it's difficult to put in ten minutes of exercise. But remember, exercise is your priority—ten minutes a day even when you're away from home.

The Banquet (Short) Circuit

I admit there may be times when following the 30-day diet will not be easy. You get trapped staring at food you know you shouldn't have. The banquet circuit is a prime example. You can avoid all the embarrassment (and hunger pangs) of turning down dinner by planning ahead and requesting a vegetarian dish or fish. I'd be surprised if your host wouldn't accommodate you.

But what if you can't plan ahead or your host couldn't accommodate your request? Trust me, you can still survive. All you have to do is eat the vegetables and the salad. You can even eat the bread—just don't put butter on it. If fish is being served, you're in luck—as long as the fish isn't bathed in cream sauce. Also, pass on the dessert. After all, you'll hardly be missing anything anyway. We all know banquet meals are rarely memorable. Of course, you'll most likely leave the place hungry. So, just do what I do. Stop at an all-night supermarket on the way home and pick up some fresh fruit.

"Oh, But I'm So Hungry!"

I can read your thoughts now. "That's fine advice. But what am I going to do *until* I get to the supermarket? My stomach is churning, the meeting is boring, the vegetables were mushy; I'm *starving*! Besides, the dessert looks wonderful."

It's difficult, I know. I've been there. I've sat there ready to lecture to a thousand people on the benefits of diet and exercise, having skipped most of the meal, and then been faced with a succulent-looking chocolate mousse. It was gorgeous, and I wanted to dig right into it. Being hungry made it even harder to resist. It's tough to stick to a diet at times like this. It's even tougher when you're a diet doctor who is a fitness fanatic. Everyone watches to see if *you'll* eat the chocolate mousse! So, having human taste buds, too, I understand how hard it is. But I've turned it down (and I don't even need to lose weight!), so I know you can do it. Eventually you'll learn to bring apples with you and leave them in the car. Better yet, eat an apple or two just before you go to the banquet.

Blow the Meal, But Not the Diet

I realize there are times when you'll go off the diet; it just can't be helped. You might go to a business lunch at a client's favorite restaurant, where he or she insists you have the chef's salad, which has plenty of cheese and dressing. You know it's off the diet and contains too many calories, but it's important not to risk insulting and possibly losing the client. So go ahead and eat it. But you must compensate. How? Get right back on track at

EXERCISE—THE ANTI-STRESS FORMULA

Does a spat with the boss put a knot between your shoulder blades? Does the thought of putting in ten hours of work in a five-hour time slot cause your back to tense and heart to pound?

Such things are signs of stress—a too-common response to the demands of the modern-day business world.

There is no easy way to combat the stress that goes along with a job, but there is an easy way to relieve the muscle tension that can result from its everyday annoyances.

Simply take some time out to relax. Shake those anxious thoughts from your head and go through this series of stress-reducing exercises. I guarantee, you'll be able to feel the tension leave your body.

1. Stand or sit erect with your chin tucked in close to your chest. Turn your head slowly to the right, trying to bring your chin over your right shoulder. Hold for three seconds. Rotate your head back to the center position. Pause. Repeat in the opposite direction. Repeat the entire sequence five times.

2. Push your chin downward, trying to touch it to your chest, without causing too much strain. Pause. Slowly lift your head and lean it backward as far as possible, again without straining. Pause. Repeat five times.

3. Bend your head slowly to the right, trying to bring your right ear to your shoulder. Pause. Return slowly to the center position. Pause. Repeat in the opposite direction. Repeat the sequence five times.

4. Slowly roll your head clockwise in as wide a circle as possible for three complete circles. Repeat in a counterclockwise motion. Pause. Repeat the sequence three times.

5. Stand erect, arms held loosely by your sides. Breathe deeply as you lift your shoulders first as high and then as far back as they will move. Breathe out as you lower your shoulders to the starting position and relax.

the next meal (don't wait until tomorrow), and stick with salads, fruits and vegetables until you feel you've paid your "dues." It's okay to slip backward every now and then if you compensate by eating less at your next meal. You'll be able to catch up and continue toward your fat-loss goal.

This also applies to exercise. I realize there will be days when you can't exercise because of travel and business, but those are rare if you're honest with yourself. So when they do happen, double up on exercise either the day before or the day after. Don't go two days in a row without exercise. Even only five minutes of exercise is better than none at all.

Before you know it (and after some trial and error), following good eating and exercise habits will become second nature to you, even while you're on business trips or entertaining a client.

Repeat 20 times, at least twice a day. Build up this routine to 50 times, twice a day.

6. Sit erect. Place your hands on your shoulders. Try to cross your elbows by bringing your right arm to the left and left arm to the right, until you feel the stretch across your upper back. Return to the starting position, drop your hands and relax. Repeat ten times.

7. Hold a one-to-two-pound weight in one hand (anything you can easily handle will do). Bending your knees slightly, bend forward at the waist and grab the end of a table with the other hand. Allow your weighted arm to dangle freely. Swing your arm laterally across your body (from the right and the left) for one minute, keeping your elbow perfectly straight. Next swing your arm backward and forward for one minute. Then swing your arm in a gradually increasing circle clockwise for one minute. Repeat counterclockwise. Change arms and repeat. Do the entire sequence three times.

8. Lie on your back with your arms above your head and your knees bent. Bring one knee as far as possible toward your chest and at the same time straighten out the other leg. Return to your original position and repeat the movements, switching legs. Relax. Repeat the exercise three times.

9. Lie on your back with a small pillow under your head, your arms at your sides and your knees bent. Bring your knees to your chest and, with clasped hands, pull your knees toward your chest. Hold for a count of ten, keeping your knees together and your shoulders flat on the floor. Repeat the pulling and holding movement three times. Relax. Repeat the exercise three times.

10. Sit in a straight-backed chair with your arms folded loosely in front of you. Let your body drop until your head is down between your knees. Pull your body back up into a sitting position while tightening your abdominal muscles. Relax. Repeat the exercise three times.

Chapter 8
ESPECIALLY FOR WOMEN

Personal beauty is a better introduction than any letter of recommendation.

— Aristotle

"I was a fat teenager. If you're a young girl and you're overweight, this can be pretty traumatic, as it's a really important time in your life. Other children make fun of you and the boys can make it even more difficult for you. It's a sad situation. You think this is the way you'll be for the rest of your life. It's really very depressing."

This is the way one 30-year-old patient summed up her youth as she sat in my office 100 pounds thinner for the first time in 15 years. She was a brand-new person and *very* proud of herself. And so was I.

"You know, before I came to see you, I only managed to lose 20 or 30 pounds at a shot. Then I'd gain it back."

Says another patient, "I lost the same 10 or 20 pounds for years. Every time I'd gain it back I'd just add a few more pounds."

Society has placed tremendous pressure on women to appear as glamorous and svelte as television and magazine models. Consequently, whether it's Cheryl Tiegs, Christina Ferrare or Christy Brinkley, there's a certain envy in every woman's eye as she critically views these beautiful women.

Over the last five years I've noticed a startling increase in the number of letters that I receive from overweight women, particularly teenage girls. And the number of young girls with anorexia (self-starvation) and bulimia (self-induced vomiting) that I see at my Institute has increased tenfold. Frankly, I find it frightening. To my mind, the search for this toothpicklike image has gotten way out of hand. Even *regular* dieting is usually extreme, mainly because too many people go about it so badly. They sacrifice their health in the process.

More than 75 percent of the patients that I treat for weight control are women in quest of a thinner body. In talking to them I find that I am usually not their first resort for weight-loss aid—I'm their last. Before me have come the whole gamut of fad diets—all characterized by too little food, or even worse, near-starvation, followed by rapid weight loss. Then in a few short weeks they gain the weight back and start the cycle over again. If any of them try exercise at all, they have to give it up because their undernourished bodies simply lack the energy to get them to move. As I said, I find this frightening. Why? Because this type of dieting, known as the yo-yo syndrome, is about the worst thing you can do to your body.

Skinny, But Fat

Yo-yo dieting has a devastating effect on the body's muscle-fat ratio. Each time you go on a diet you lose more muscle mass and every time you gain back the weight you gain back more fat. Keep it up for a long period of time and you end up a skinny but flabby person. Take, for example, a 21-year-old who weighs 120 pounds and has 20 percent body fat. If she spends the next five years yo-yoing between the 120 and 140 pounds, she may end up 120 pounds again at age 26, but she'll also end up with a lot more body fat and a lot less muscle than she had at age 21. Why? Yo-yo dieting has altered her body composition. And the condition will get worse as she gets older because the body's ability to replace lean body mass will decrease with each decade of her life.

One of the reasons this happens is that the body rebels when it is deprived of food. Starving the cells of nourishment only trains them to adjust to a lower calorie intake, which means that your metabolism slows down. The other reason is lack of exercise. A body that's revved up to go turns to fat rather than lean body tissue for fuel. So exercise actually protects lean body tissue and attacks fat. This isn't a theory; there's scientific evidence to prove it.

In one study, a group of people were put on a 1,000-calorie-a-day diet. Half were put on an exercise regimen and the other half were instructed not to exercise at all. After seven weeks, the nonexercisers lost an average of 18 pounds—7 pounds' worth of lean body tissue and 11 pounds of fat. The exercised group, for all their effort, lost only 1 pound more, an average of 19 pounds. However, they only lost 4 pounds of lean body tissue. An impressive 15 pounds was fat.

The moral to the story is this: Sensible and gradual weight loss coupled with a regular exercise program is your *only* route to a beautiful body. Stop looking for shortcuts.

Exercise Doesn't Masculinize Women

I tell women all the time that exercise is nothing but *good* for them. That they *must* exercise. But I have to admit (and this goes for men, too) that I do run into my share of resisters. That's because there's still a contingent of women out there who are under the misguided notion that exercise will only make them look muscular. They're afraid they'll end up losing their femininity. Nothing could be farther from the truth.

There is a major difference between men and women in the way they increase muscle mass and decrease body fat. The muscle-bound look that men attain is a direct result of the male hormone, testosterone. And 99 percent of all women do not have an adequate amount of testosterone to make them look like a Charlene Atlas. A woman who takes up weight training or exercise will simply define the muscles she has and help them to function more efficiently. She will gradually replace the fat in her arms and legs with more well-toned muscles.

It's important for women to realize that regular exercise will increase their muscle mass and reduce their body fat, but it will not masculinize them. It will simply make them more shapely.

Also, more muscle and less fat also means a more efficient use of calories because muscles burn calories faster than fat. That alone is reason enough to shave fat in favor of muscle! For instance, a woman who is very muscular and weighs 115 pounds can eat more calories to maintain her weight than a woman of the same weight who is "spongier" due to more body fat.

Look Younger, Feel Younger

A routine exercise program and a healthy diet can do wonders for any woman's appearance. Take a mental inventory of everyone in your neighborhood or workplace of approximately the same age. Are there some who look better than others? Are there some who defy their years? Of course there are. And I'd make a wager that those who look younger than their age are active people who exercise and eat properly.

Why am I so sure of this? Because for most of my career I've watched people seemingly grow younger as they've taken up exercise and a more healthy lifestyle.

"I look better than I've looked in ten years," say some. "I look better than I've looked in my life," say even more.

These types of comments are more than personal opinions. There's actually a scientific reason for the improvement.

The right combination of exercise and diet provides the tissues of your body with the best nourishment possible and provides more oxygen to those tissues, thereby preventing decay. Studies have also shown that exercisers have thicker skin than nonexercisers, which helps contribute to an exerciser's youthful appearance. The result: a younger-looking you.

The Way to Beautiful Breasts

If exercise can tone your arms and legs, is it also capable of toning your breasts? Well, not exactly. But it can tone the underlying muscles and improve the breasts' contour and shape.

Since breasts are composed of fatty tissue, glands and ligaments, they cannot increase in size through exercise as muscles do. Muscles, such as the upper pectorals which fill out the inner portion (cleavage area) of your breasts, can be developed through weight training. Since the pectoral muscles are two triangular muscles attached across the top of the chest down along the sternum and under the arm diagonally across the rib cage, they can enhance the contour of the breast when developed. In fact, these muscles will be the most significant in contributing to an improved breast appearance. Weight training can improve the appearance of the breasts by increasing not only the size of the muscles, but the tone of the muscles surrounding the breast tissue.

Most experts agree that after six to eight weeks of weight training, a significant difference in breast appearance will be noted, and that after 12 months a dramatic improvement will be obvious.

So don't believe the false claims that are often advertised in magazines suggesting instant breast enlargement. The only instant breast enlargements are silicone implants provided by cosmetic surgeons.

But even the size of the breasts is not as important as the symmetrical development that weight training can provide.

In addition to improving the appearance of your breasts, weight training or isometrics can strengthen and tone the supporting muscles of the breasts, preventing sagging and other aging effects caused by gravity.

The best weight-training exercise for developing pectoral muscles is the bench press. In fact, sets of 12 to 15 with a weight that you can tolerate is the best routine. Most routines should consist of 3 to 5 sets depending upon the amount of weight that you're lifting.

BUST DEVELOPING YOU CAN DO AT HOME

If weight training's not your style, or if you simply don't have the time or money to participate in a planned program, there is still plenty you can do to contour your breasts. Do the following exercises (all of which can be done in the privacy of your home) 5 times at first, building up to 25 times 3 to 5 times a day. You should notice improvement in about eight weeks. Remember, you're probably using muscles that you haven't used in quite some time. Therefore, expect some minor aches and pains in the early stages of the program.

• Push-ups. Do them any way you possibly can. As your arms develop and your chest muscles become stronger you'll be able to do them properly.

• Hold two ten-pound cans of vegetables or fruit in your hands and stand erect facing the mirror. Now extend your arms directly out in front of you, then extend your arms away from your chest. Bring your arms together. Repeat.

• Lie flat on your back on a bench and, holding two ten-pound cans, extend your arms above you and then gently lower your arms to your chest. Straighten your arms and repeat.

Here is the weight-training routine for breast development that I suggest to the women who come to my institute:
• Develop a series of upper-body exercises with light weights at 12 to 15 repetitions. Do 3 sets every other day.
• Emphasize bench-pressing exercises.
• Do 10 to 20 push-ups a day.
• Do 10 to 20 pull-ups a day.
• Do the following isometric exercises daily: Clasp hands together in front of you and press one against the other, holding for 15 seconds. Repeat several times.

The Universal Concern: Cellulite

"I've tried everything to lose that extra fat in my thighs, but nothing seemed to work. My mother and sister both have big thighs; it's simply a family trait," lamented my patient.

In fact, she had tried everything, but to no avail—fasting, electrical stimulation, herbal wraps, you name it—in hopes of ridding herself of cellulite deposits on the hips, buttocks, thighs and abdomen. Some experts claim there's simply no way of getting rid of cellulite once you've got it. I don't agree. You can significantly reduce the amount (I won't claim you can get rid of all of it) through exercise. I'm not going to kid you and tell you it's easy to get rid of. It isn't. But by following a good aerobic program, you should start seeing results in 90 days. It just takes that long to mobilize fat deposits from those problem areas.

A good rule of thumb for weight loss in women is that inches go first, pounds second and cellulite third. So hang in there, for you need not be plagued with "saddlebag syndrome" forever. And no one is beyond hope; it simply takes longer in some people than others to lose those unwanted dimples.

Most experts agree that exercise will reduce your body fat and prevent the number of fat cells from increasing. In addition, research has suggested that empty fat cells may even prevent new fat cells from being formed. So I'd suggest aerobic exercise—walking, jogging, bicycling, swimming and so on—daily for the next 90 days in order to get results. In addition, a low-fat and high-fiber diet can only help speed things along.

A Little Help from a Friend

"Okay," you say. "I'm convinced. But the house needs to be cleaned, the children need to be fed, the dog has to be walked and I have a full-time job. Where am I supposed to find the time to exercise?"

You can start by making exercise—and yourself—your first priority. Once you realize the need for this and make the commitment to yourself, you won't have any trouble finding the time. If you must, let something else suffer, like the housework or shopping. But not your health.

Without knowing specific circumstances, I can only offer some suggestions. If the problem is children, find another woman who's interested in fitness and involve her in your exercise program. She can babysit while you exercise, then you can babysit while she exercises.

If you can't find anyone, hire a babysitter while you exercise. I know it will cost some money, but the returns are worth it.

Okay, you can't find anyone to trade off babysitting and you don't want to hire a babysitter or can't find someone you trust? Well, don't give up yet.

Buy yourself a stationary bike. If money is a problem, try a garage sale. You'll find one at the right price–somewhere. Then, while the children sleep, set it up in front of the television and ride while you watch your favorite show, read or talk on the phone.

Get your husband or boyfriend involved and exercise together. You have one lifestyle together, why not *change* lifestyles together? When he gets home at night, instead of having cocktails, hand him his exercise clothes and go for a run or walk. If that doesn't work, set the alarm a little earlier in the morning so that the two of you can exercise before you begin your day.

If you can involve him, you'll see it helps a lot. You'll both be following the diet (no fixing two meals), you'll both be exercising. When one feels lazy, the other can become the motivator.

This program of couples working together can make a big difference. In fact, two of my exemplary patients who were Mollenized together are Kathy and David.

"Before starting the Mollen Method I'd never been able to lose weight successfully. I'd lost weight before on fad diets and always gained it right back real fast. I enjoy the walking. When I started walking, I started feeling better. It's easier to do it together like this. I'm not one to exercise alone," said Kathy.

"As for the diet, we ate no red meat. We ate fish probably every night and a lot of vegetables, but the main thing is we started learning about calories," said David. "It was great to have my wife cooking and eating the same foods that I needed in order to lose weight."

So Kathy lost 22 pounds in six weeks and David lost more than 30 pounds in eight weeks, when neither one had ever been successful at losing weight and keeping it off in the past.

"It's been a tremendous help doing it together," said Kathy.

"I can't imagine it working if both people are not involved. It would take a very strong will," said David.

Losing weight together makes sense for other reasons. As Kathy explains, "I think it works for us because we're together. We have each other to talk to about it. You can be proud of each other. If you are doing it alone, you might have a bad day and eat food you shouldn't or skip the exercise. But if your mate also is involved in the Mollen Method, the support and understanding will help you overcome the bad days."

So get your mate and get started. You'll be glad you did.

Beverly's Remarkable Finish

When it comes to stories about giving it your all there is none in my experience which outdoes the story of Beverly Steen. I met Beverly the night prior to a marathon in Globe, Arizona. I was the featured speaker, and I planned to run the marathon together with Beverly's father, who was a patient of mine. A 10K (6.2 mile) run was scheduled to start at the same time as the marathon, and this was the race that Beverly had planned to enter. Beverly, 21 years old at the time, told me how she'd been running six miles daily for the past six months in preparation for it.

As the evening progressed I tried convincing Beverly that she should run the marathon instead of the 10K, as I thought that she was appropriately prepared to cover the distance. She was quite skeptical, however, as well as unsure of herself. Her remarks were, "Do you really think I can do it? I'm not prepared and I am so nervous. I can't imagine running 26 miles without killing myself." At the evening's end she said she'd think about it and decide in the morning whether she'd run the marathon or not.

As the sun rose over the mountain for the start of the First Annual Globe Marathon, Beverly also rose for her first marathon. She ran with her father and myself for the first half and then suddenly proclaimed, "I feel great, I think I'll pick up my pace for awhile." I told her to be careful not to go too fast as she might hit the proverbial "wall" and not finish.

As Beverly's father and I continued along our way, I told him that she probably wouldn't finish because her increased pace would only wear her out. In fact, we slowed our pace because it was extremely warm. We never spotted Beverly again during the marathon and wondered whether she had to stop and been picked up by one of the aid station vehicles.

When we crossed the finish line there was Beverly, absolutely exhilarated. I asked with concern, "Did you finish? How do you feel?" Beverly replied, "Great, I won!"

As I recovered from my shock, she told me how she'd passed all other women at the 20-mile mark and they had never caught up to her again.

The moral of this story is that if you have confidence, you can do anything you want to.

Exercise and Pregnancy

I've been motivating women to lose weight and get in shape for the past 15 years, and I take great pride in watching their accomplishments. I'm particularly proud to see them turn into happy individuals, especially when they come bounding through the door with "Guess what, I'm pregnant!" Unfortunately, though, after the elation wears off (or the baby is born), they end up back in my office with one big concern: "Will I ever get thin again?"

"Of course," I tell them. In fact, a body in shape before pregnancy is easier to get back in shape after pregnancy. It's the out-of-shape women who must struggle to lose pounds after a baby is born. In fact, I think any woman who wants to have a baby should consider it her duty to get in shape before she gets pregnant. It's best both for her and her baby. Recent research has suggested that a healthy body will not only conceive more easily, but it will protect the fetus and present fewer risks to the baby after conception.

The average woman gains 25 to 30 pounds during pregnancy. It's important that the prospective mother-to-be keep her weight under control, since an overweight woman increases the risk of complications during pregnancy.

Most aerobic exercises, such as walking, bicycling, swimming, aerobic dancing and even jogging, offer benefits and minimal risk to the would-be mother prior to pregnancy. The easiest way to get in shape before conception is to walk, bicycle or swim daily starting with 10 minutes and building up to 30 minutes daily over three months' time.

Exercises that strengthen the abdominal muscles (such as sit-ups and leg raises) can provide the would-be mother more support for her abdominal organs and reduce the stress and pressure on her lower back, which develop as the spine gradually changes its position during pregnancy. As a result, many pregnant women complain of lower back pain, especially during the latter stages of pregnancy.

For the woman concerned about developing varicose veins in her legs during pregnancy, improving the tone and strength of the legs prior to conception will reduce the chances considerably.

Almost every woman is concerned about her breasts stretching and sagging as a result of pregnancy. A way to prevent this is to develop and strengthen the pectoral muscles below the breast tissue. These will help to hold up the breasts and take some of the stress off supporting ligament tissue.

Controlling your weight will help to prevent your breast size from significantly increasing, as excess fatty tissue commonly deposits in the breasts. Just as weight control is important in preventing sagging breasts after pregnancy, it is also important in preventing stretch marks on the abdomen, breasts and buttocks.

The woman who is 50 pounds overweight and plans to conceive is jeopardizing not only her health, but the future health of her baby. Since

BENEFITS OF EXERCISE DURING PREGNANCY

By getting in shape before and staying in shape during pregnancy, you'll be able to reap the following benefits:

- Weight control
- Improved digestion
- Better sleeping patterns
- Less anxiety and frustration
- Healthier baby

- Fewer obstetrical complications
- Fewer stretch marks
- Increased muscle tone
- Quicker fat loss and regained body shape after pregnancy

obesity is a contributing risk factor to diabetes, high blood pressure and toxemia during pregnancy, any woman who is 20 or more pounds over-weight should get in shape by losing weight and exercising for at least 90 days before she attempts to conceive.

Finally, the most important advice I can offer to would-be mothers is to stop smoking and drinking alcohol *before* conception. Recent research has suggested that women who smoke have a much higher risk of sponta-neous abortions and babies with lower birth weights than women who do not smoke. In addition, a report in the *Journal of the American Medical Association* suggests that there is no safe amount of alcohol consumption during pregnancy. Therefore, try to stop drinking and smoking before conceiving as it will be much harder to stop once you're pregnant.

If you were an exerciser before pregnancy, you most likely can con-tinue to exercise once you've become pregnant. Just make sure you get an okay from your doctor. As you get closer to full term you'll probably have to cut back on your exercise because of the physical aspects of carrying the baby.

Last but not least, make sure you eat properly during your pregnancy. A low-fat diet with plenty of fruits and vegetables that emphasizes low salt and no caffeine—in fact, the Mollen Method—is about the best a mother-to-be can do for her body.

Unfortunately, many overweight women believe pregnancy is a great time for "open season on food." Just remember, if it wasn't good for you when you weren't pregnant, it certainly can't be any good for you when you are. So, be sensible—eat sensibly.

Chapter 9

SEX, PASSION AND FITNESS

Fitness is sexy because it's about bodies. It's about moving and sweating; about thighs and hips and buttocks and arms; about getting stronger and firmer. But sexy is one thing and sex—making love—is another. Sure, working out can make you sexier. But can it also make you have more—and better—sex?

Well, there's no blanket rule (pardon the pun). But I think the Mollen Method can improve your sex life. And so do my patients.

"My sex life has improved 100 percent since I started the Mollen Method" is how one of them put it. "I can't believe how sexy my husband thinks I am. And I respond better to him because I feel better about myself."

That 100 percent increase probably had more to do with the *quality* of her sex life than the *quantity*. Yet some experts suggest that exercisers *do* have more sex. A study conducted by Lawrence Katzman, Ph.D., a sex educator and counselor here in Phoenix, showed that fit men had more sexual desire and a better attitude about sex than men who were out of shape. What's more, his study found that physically active men in their late forties and fifties had sex as frequently as the younger men in the study. Now that should make you guys lace up your running shoes!

(And that's just what Dr. Katzman tells his patients to do. Along with counseling, he believes that exercise is the best prescription for problems like impotence, lack of desire, premature ejaculation or an inability to achieve orgasm.)

Why does the Mollen Method improve your sex life? First off, it makes you healthier. And when you're free of the aches and pains that tag along with sickness you're more likely to think of the bed as a place for fun rather than recuperation. Second, sexual desire—yours and your partner's—is heightened when your body is well toned and firm. But it's not only the physical changes that do the trick. It's the mental changes, too.

If you're 20 pounds overweight, for instance, you may not feel worthy of being touched or caressed. That feeling, especially if it's unexpressed, can make your partner feel rejected. A poor self image can even sabotage your orgasm; after all, you don't deserve to feel pleasure.

When you exercise, you become more aware of yourself—of who you are and what you can do. This lets you deal with people more positively and with more energy; you feel good about yourself so you feel good about the people around you. In the sexual realm, this interpersonal sensitivity translates into more hugs, touching, kissing and caressing. One of my patients says it best: "The emotional and sexual fulfillment I received from the Mollen Method are indescribable."

Maybe so, but let me give it a whirl starting with how exercise might improve your marriage.

Bed and Bored

Many couples would rather turn on the TV than each other. They used to be filled with desire, but the years drained their passion. They have sex—sometimes—but it's by the numbers. About as exciting as reading the dictionary. Or a little less.

Why? Why does sex in marriage become routine or nonexistent? Well, there could be lots of reasons. But I know one that's common. One or both partners have become—let's face it—unattractive. They've gained weight, and flab isn't a turn-on. Let Pat tell you about her experience in this area.

"For ten years, my sex life was dead. And buried. I mean *nothing*. I was 100 pounds overweight, and my husband found me ... well, unattractive, to say the least. He claimed he simply couldn't have sex with someone that overweight. I always thought that if you really loved somebody, you could overlook their body and still show some kind of love. But not him. In fact, even after I lost 50 pounds he didn't show me any physical affection. I even started thinking about getting it from someone else, and that's pretty sad."

Fortunately, Pat did lost 100 pounds—and regained her husband's attentions. But now that she's thin, how would she feel about an overweight spouse?

"I can sympathize with my husband more now—I wouldn't want a mate who was 50 pounds overweight now that I'm thin."

It would be great if we could love and desire our spouses no matter what, but we're just not put together that way. There's still the animal in us that wants someone who excites us, who's vital and energetic – and lean. In fact, I think that a marriage itself could be said to be "out of shape" when one or both partners get that way.

Overweight isn't the only thing that sinks sex. Age does too. But there's no reason it should.

Young at Heart – and Every Other Part

Hot: It's the modern term for sexy. Well, getting older doesn't have to mean getting colder. In fact, many people report active sex lives well into their eighties. For some of them, the secret is *fitness*.

Like Dimitri Iordonis, a Greek marathon runner who finished the race in 7 hours, 40 minutes. True, at that pace he could have been lapped by a world-class runner – but Dimitri was 96 years old at the time. After the race, the press interviewed him to find out how he stayed so spry just short of the century mark.

"I gave up alcohol, tobacco, red meats and fat," he said.

"Anything else?" asked one reporter.

"I gave up sex at age 90."

Perhaps you won't give up sex until 90, either. You can tell the reporter it's because you followed the Mollen Method.

Everything You Always Wanted to Know about Sex and Fitness – But Were Too Out of Shape to Ask

I write a syndicated column called, "The Art of Feeling Good." Many of my readers write to ask me questions, and a lot of those questions are about sex and exercise. Since there seems to be so much confusion about this subject, I'd like to share some of the questions – and the answers – with you.

"I have a rather unusual question," one woman wrote to me. "Your column on fitness enhancing sexuality definitely applies to me – I exercise for one hour every day and I have a strong sex drive. I could make love for an hour every day, too. But my husband's exercise habits are minimal – and so is his sex drive. Is there any way to reduce mine other than becoming overweight, stopping exercise, masturbating or committing adultery? They are terrible alternatives. Help!"

I wrote back advising her to be honest with her husband: "Tell him, 'Hey, look, I'm exercising regularly. I feel better about myself, more sexual and physical. So I need you to exercise and get in shape!'" Tell him right up front, I said, that you think exercise is essential for your relationship to survive.

I don't think this woman's problem is a rarity. In fact, it's why I always encourage couples to exercise together. And even if a mate says no to exercise at first, your success in losing weight and looking better may be just the spark he or she needs to get started.

Here's another letter from one of my readers on a question that's enshrined in locker-room mythology: Will sex before an athletic event drain energy?

"My husband is 35 years old and plays softball for his company," said the reader. "He's a fair player, but he had never hit a home run in his life. Last weekend we made love in the afternoon—right before his game. He hit *three* home runs!"

Well, I don't think this is the last word on the subject, but I also think that pre-event intercourse isn't harmful, and may even be helpful. (After all, it decreases tension, and jitters are a frequent cause of athletic failure.)

A Run-Down Sex Life

Okay, I've spent a lot of time trying to convince you that exercise revs up your sex drive. But some people think just the opposite—that exercise drains you, so that you don't have energy for sex. Even a study in *MD Magazine* reported that people who jog 25 to 100 miles a week may experience a decrease in libido (that's the scientific name for sex drive).

Is this true?

I hate to say it, but . . . in a few cases it might be. Those few cases are (1) marathon runners who (2) increase their training mileage by 50 miles per week. You might be saying to yourself: Of course, they're too *tired* for sex. And you'd be right—that's exactly what one study showed. All that extra running—or excessive exercise of any kind—may also decrease the levels of testosterone, the male hormone.

So for the typical exerciser, this problem is practically nonexistent. Just as I've been telling you, it's the opposite "problem" that you'll have to deal with—a stronger sex drive.

Is Sex Exercise?

Yes, but it's a 50-yard dash, not a mile run. Intercourse usually lasts from 5 to 20 minutes, and during that time your pulse doesn't speed up too much–except right before and during orgasm. Then it's around 150; high enough, but unfortunately not long enough, for a conditioning effect. (If it was, there's no doubt which "aerobic exercise" most of the population would choose. And people like me wouldn't have to harp on the daily exercise requirement, either.) Also, calories burned during sex usually don't total more than 30 to 60.

For certain people, though, even the minor exertion of sex can seem like an ultramarathon: heart attack victims. But notice that I said *seem.* A better word might be *imagine.* It's fear that stops heart patients from having sex, not reality. Sex really doesn't call on the heart to pump extra hard, and studies show that recovering heart attack victims can resume sexual activities quickly. (Of course, check with your doctor.) It's interesting to note that exercise improves their sex life too: Heart attack patients who start an exercise program can usually resume sex sooner than patients who don't exercise.

Exercise–The Ultimate Aphrodisiac

We've tried almost everything. Pulverized rhino horn. Oysters. Ginseng. If it could turn up the lust level, folks have swallowed it, sniffed it, smoked it–even bathed in it. But there's something unsavory about this quest for the ultimate aphrodisiac, or *any* aphrodisiac. Particularly since the real thing is right at hand–or at foot. Exercise.

What type of exercise is best for improving your sex life? I think you already know the answer: aerobic. Walking, jogging, bicycling, swimming, aerobic dancing–anything that gets your heart pumping and keeps it pumping for 30 minutes or so. These exercises increase your endurance, including your sexual stamina.

Now you may think that I don't know that sex also has something to do with love. But don't get me wrong. I'm a romantic; I even believe in love at first sight. Only it's more than love that starts the heart pounding. It's a kind of aura, an impression of sensuality, an inviting radiance: the glow of good looks and good health. Love, I think, has its basis in that physical attraction. And if that feeling isn't there, it's next to impossible to create. Exercise will help: It's loving yourself and helping others love you.

Chapter 10
RECIPES

Ambrosia Medley

Yields: approximately 3 cups
Serving size: ¾ cup
Calories per serving: 95

- 1 cup (½ pint) strawberries, halved
- 1 cup fresh or canned (juice-packed) pineapple tidbits
- 1 medium banana, sliced
- ¼ cup unsweetened flaked coconut
- ⅓ cup orange juice

Combine strawberries, pineapple and bananas in a large bowl. Sprinkle with coconut. Drizzle with orange juice. Chill before serving.

Art's Brown Apple

My favorite dessert.

Yields: approximately 3 cups
Serving size: 1 cup
Calories per serving: 140

- 1 cup fresh bread crumbs
- ⅓ cup wheat bran
- 3 tablespoons margarine, melted
- 3 cups (3 to 4 medium) sliced apples
- ¼ cup honey
- 2 tablespoons water
- ½ teaspoon cinnamon
  - Dash of nutmeg
- ½ teaspoon grated lemon peel
  - Juice of 1 lemon
- 1½ teaspoons margarine (20% diet only)

Combine bread crumbs, bran and margarine in a small bowl and set aside.

In a large bowl, mix together apples, honey, water, cinnamon, nutmeg, lemon peel and half of the lemon juice.

Spray a 2-quart casserole with non-stick spray and layer a third of the bread crumb mixture, then half of the apple mixture. Repeat layering, then sprinkle with remaining third of bread crumbs. Drizzle remaining lemon juice over top. If following 20 percent diet, dot with margarine.

Cover and bake in preheated 350°F oven for 20 minutes.

Asparagus Delight

Yields: approximately 2 cups
Serving size: ½ cup
Calories per serving: 16

  ½ cup water
  1 tablespoon chopped onions
  1 tablespoon chopped green peppers
  1 teaspoon chopped pimientos
      (optional)
      Dash of pepper
  1½ cups (10-ounce package) frozen
      asparagus spears or cut asparagus
  1 teaspoon tarragon vinegar or cider
      vinegar

In a medium-size saucepan, bring water, onions, green peppers, pimientos and pepper to a boil. Add asparagus; bring to a boil. Simmer, covered, until tender, about 5 minutes. Drain asparagus. Sprinkle with vinegar and serve.

Banana Pop

Yields: 2 pops
Serving size: 1 pop
Calories per serving: 60

  1 medium banana
  1 tablespoon toasted wheat germ

Peel banana and cut in half cross-wise. Gently insert wooden sticks into cut ends of banana halves and roll them in wheat germ. Stand pops in a jar and freeze.

Buttermilk Dressing

Yields: 1 cup
Serving size: 1 tablespoon
Calories per serving: 6

  1 cup buttermilk
  1½ teaspoons vinegar
  1¼ teaspoons dillweed
  ¼ teaspoon minced garlic
      Freshly ground pepper to taste

Combine buttermilk, vinegar, dill-weed, garlic and pepper in a blender and process until thoroughly mixed. Chill.

Carrot-Orange Toss

Serve this as a salad or a dessert.

Yields: approximately 3 cups
Serving size: ½ cup
Calories per serving: 100

  2 medium navel oranges, peeled and
      diced
  2 cups grated carrots
  ½ cup raisins
  2 tablespoons honey
  1 teaspoon lemon juice
  12 large lettuce leaves

In a large bowl, combine oranges, carrots, raisins, honey and lemon juice. Chill.

Place ½ cup of mixture on 2 lettuce leaves and serve.

Cheesy Potatoes

Yields: 1½ to 2 cups
Serving size: 1 cup
Calories per serving: 190

    4 cups water
    2 medium potatoes, quartered
    1 ounce low-fat cheese (any kind)
      Dash of nutmeg

In a medium-size saucepan, bring water to a boil. Add potatoes. Cook, covered, over medium heat for 15 to 20 minutes, or until tender.

Drain potatoes. Peel and dice.

Spray an 8-by-8-inch shallow baking dish with nonstick spray. Spread potatoes in the dish, layering them evenly (layers should not be too thick). Tear cheese into small pieces and sprinkle on top. Sprinkle with nutmeg.

Place potatoes under broiler and cook for 5 minutes, or until cheese is bubbly and lightly brown on top.

Chicken Kabobs

Serve singly as an hors d'oeuvre or 3 kabobs as a meal (102 calories).

Yields: 12 kabobs
Serving size: 1 kabob
Calories per serving: 34

    1 whole boneless chicken breast, cut
      into 24 pieces, skin and fat removed
    1 medium green pepper, cut into 24
      pieces
    1 medium apple, cored and cut into
      24 pieces

    1 teaspoon lemon juice
    1 tablespoon apple juice
    1 teaspoon lemon pepper

On each of 12 skewers alternate 1 piece of chicken, green pepper and apple. Repeat once.

In a small bowl, combine lemon juice, apple juice and lemon pepper. Set aside.

Broil kabobs for 4 to 5 minutes on each side, basting midway with juice mixture.

Chicken Pocket Sandwiches

Yields: 2 sandwiches
Serving size: 1 sandwich
Calories per serving: 284

    1 cup chopped cabbage
    ¾ cup diced cooked chicken
    ½ cup chopped carrots
    ¼ cup chopped radishes
    ½ cup plain, low-fat yogurt
    2 tablespoons skim milk
    1 teaspoon prepared mustard
    ¼ teaspoon crushed dried thyme
    2 pita bread rounds, halved
    ¼ cup shredded low-fat Cheddar cheese

In a medium bowl, combine cabbage, chicken, carrots and radishes and set aside.

In a small bowl, combine yogurt, milk, mustard and thyme. Stir into cabbage mixture; chill.

Spoon mixture into bread halves. Sprinkle cheese on top and serve.

Chilled Shrimp and Mushroom Kabobs

Yields: 3 kabobs
Serving size: 1 kabob
Calories per serving: 200

- ¼ pound whole fresh mushrooms, stems removed
- ½ medium cucumber, peeled, quartered, and cut into chunks
- ½ pound cooked shrimp, peeled and cleaned
- 1½ tablespoons safflower or corn oil
- 1 tablespoon white or cider vinegar
- ½ cup diced onions
- 1 tablespoon lemon juice
- 1 tablespoon water
- 2 teaspoons prepared horseradish
  Pepper to taste
- ¼ teaspoon garlic powder
  Dash of dried tarragon
- 12 cherry tomatoes

Place mushroom caps in a large bowl with cucumber chunks and shrimp.

In a small bowl, beat oil with vinegar, onions, lemon juice, water, horseradish, pepper, garlic powder and tarragon. Pour over mushrooms, cucumbers and shrimp; stir to mix well. Refrigerate, covered, several hours or overnight.

Drain mushrooms, cucumbers and shrimp.

To make kabobs, thread a tomato, mushroom, shrimp, mushroom, cucumber chunk, mushroom, etc. onto 3 skewers. Serve chilled.

Cottage Cheese and Cinnamon Toast

A nice change of taste for breakfast.

Serves: 1
Calories per serving: 102

- 1 slice rye bread
- 2 tablespoons low-fat cottage cheese
- ½ medium peach, sliced
  Cinnamon to taste

Lightly toast rye bread. Spread cottage cheese on toast. Top with peach slices and sprinkle with cinnamon. Place under broiler until heated through, about 4 minutes.

Cucumber-Onion Salad

Yields: 1½ cups
Serving size: ½ cup
Calories per serving: 27

- 1 cup sliced cucumber
- 1 small onion, separated into rings
- ½ cup cider vinegar or tarragon vinegar
- 1 tablespoon sugar
  Dash of pepper
- 6 lettuce leaves

Combine cucumbers, onions, vinegar, sugar and pepper in a medium-sized bowl and mix well. Chill at least 2 hours.

Drain cucumber mixture. Serve on lettuce leaves.

Cucumber Soup

A cold soup you can include in your summer menu.

Yields: approximately 2 cups
Serving size: 1 cup
Calories per serving: 55

  2 cups peeled, seeded and chopped
      cucumbers
  1 cup plain, low-fat yogurt
  1 clove garlic, crushed
  ¼ teaspoon dillweed
  ¼ teaspoon fresh mint leaves
  ¼ cup chopped scallions

In a blender or food processor, process cucumbers, yogurt, garlic, dillweed and mint until smooth. Top each 1-cup serving with 2 tablespoons scallions.

Dr. Art's Avocado Omelet

Serves: 1
Calories per serving: 157

  ⅛ avocado, diced
  ½ medium tomato, diced
  1 tablespoon plain, low-fat yogurt
  1 medium egg
  1 egg white
  1 tablespoon water
      Pepper to taste

Mix together avocados, tomatoes and yogurt in a small bowl. Set aside.

Place egg, egg white, water and pepper in a small bowl and beat lightly.

Spray an 8- or 9-inch skillet with nonstick spray and preheat. Pour egg mixture into hot skillet and tilt skillet so that mixture covers the bottom. Cook omelet over low heat until just set, 4 to 5 minutes. Spoon yogurt mixture into the center of the omelet and fold omelet in half. Serve immediately.

Fish and Vegetables à l'Orange

An easy one-dish meal.

Serves: 1
Calories per serving: 188

  ¼ teaspoon diced orange peel
  ¼ cup orange juice
  2 teaspoons soy sauce
  ¼ teaspoon grated ginger root or
      ⅛ teaspoon ground ginger
  1 medium carrot, julienned
  3 ounces codfish, tilefish or other white
      fish fillets
  ¼ cup sliced zucchini
  1 tablespoon water
  ½ teaspoon cornstarch

In a medium-size skillet, combine orange peel, orange juice, soy sauce and grated ginger root or ground ginger and cook over medium heat for 1 minute. Add carrots. Bring to a boil. Reduce heat and simmer, covered, for 5 minutes.

Push carrots to the outer edge of the skillet. Place fish in the center of the skillet. Arrange zucchini around the fish. Bring to a boil, adding more juice (if necessary), reduce heat and simmer, covered, for about 5 minutes, or until fish flakes easily when tested with a fork.

With a slotted spoon, remove fish and vegetables from the skillet and set aside.

In a small bowl, stir together water and cornstarch. Add to orange juice mixture in the skillet. Cook and stir until thickened and bubbly, about 2 minutes.

Return fish and vegetables to skillet. Heat through, spooning glaze on top. Serve immediately.

Fish Creole

Serves: 2
Calories per serving: 238

    6 ounces codfish, haddock or halibut
        fillets
    ½ tablespoon margarine
    ½ cup stewed tomatoes, coarsely
        chopped
    2 tablespoons chopped onions
    2 tablespoons diced celery
    1 tablespoon chopped green peppers
    2 tablespoons sugar
        Dash of oregano
        Dash of pepper

Arrange fish in a 9-inch square or 11 × 17-inch baking dish sprayed with nonstick spray.

In a medium-size saucepan, melt margarine. Stir in tomatoes, onions, celery, green peppers, sugar, oregano and pepper and mix well. Carefully pour tomato mixture over fish.

Bake in a preheated 350°F oven for 15 to 20 minutes, or until fish flakes easily when tested with a fork.

Fruit Ambrosia

Yields: approximately 2 cups
Serving size: ½ cup
Calories per serving: 60

    4 slices pineapple (if canned, packed in
        juice and drained), halved
    1 medium navel orange, peeled and
        sliced
    5 strawberries, halved
    1 medium banana, sliced
    ¼ cup unsweetened flaked coconut
    ¼ teaspoon allspice
        Dash of ground ginger

Arrange pineapple on the bottom of a medium-sized shallow dish. Top with oranges, strawberries, then bananas.

In a small bowl, combine coconut with allspice and ginger. Sprinkle over fruit. Chill before serving.

Fruit Blintzes

Yields: 16 blintzes
Serving size: 1 blintze
Calories per serving: 70

    1 16-ounce can juice-packed sliced
        peaches, well drained and diced
    ½ cup chopped cooked prunes
    ¾ cup skim milk
    1 cup unsifted unbleached white flour
    1 cup low-fat liquid egg substitute

In a small bowl, combine peaches and prunes and set aside.

In a large bowl, alternately add milk and flour to egg substitute, mixing until well blended.

Spray a 6-inch skillet with nonstick spray. Heat skillet. Pour a thin covering of prepared batter (about 2 tablespoons) into skillet, just enough to cover the bottom. Cook on one side until batter blisters. Turn out onto a clean cloth or wax paper. Repeat with remaining batter to make 16 blintzes, spraying pan as needed.

Place 1 tablespoonful of peach and prune mixture on each blintze. Fold in sides to form a square. Brown squares under broiler. Serve hot.

Fruit Salad Dressing

Yields: 1½ cups
Serving size: 1 tablespoon
Calories per serving: 8

 1 cup plain, low-fat yogurt
 ½ cup orange juice
 Dash of cinnamon
 2 tablespoons lemon juice

In a small bowl, combine yogurt, orange juice, cinnamon and lemon juice. Blend well.

Fruit Slush

Yields: 2 cups
Serving size: ½ cup
Calories per serving: 60

 1 16-ounce can juice-packed mixed fruit, with liquid

Place fruit with juice in a shallow 8 × 8-inch dish. Freeze until firm but not solid. Start checking it in 2 to 2½ hours.

Place frozen fruit in a blender or food processor and puree. Serve immediately.

Hearty Halibut

Serves: 2
Calories per serving: 150

 ⅓ cup thinly sliced onions
 2 3-ounce halibut steaks
 ¾ cup chopped fresh mushrooms
 2 tablespoons chopped tomatoes
 2 tablespoons chopped green peppers
 2 tablespoons chopped fresh parsley
 1½ tablespoons chopped pimientos
 ¼ cup dry white wine
 1 tablespoon lemon juice
 Dash of dillweed
 Dash of pepper
 Lemon wedges (optional)

Place onions on the bottom of an 8 × 8-inch baking dish sprayed with nonstick spray. Place fish in a single layer over onions.

In a small bowl, combine mushrooms, tomatoes, green peppers, parsley and pimientos and spread over top of fish.

In another small bowl, combine wine, lemon juice, dillweed and pepper and pour over vegetables. Bake in a preheated 350°F oven for 25 to 30 minutes, or until fish flakes easily when tested with a fork.

Serve with lemon wedges, if desired.

Italian Dressing

Yields: 1 cup
Serving size: 2 tablespoons
Calories per serving: 5

 2 tablespoons vinegar
 ⅔ cup tomato juice
 2-ounce package dry Italian dressing mix

In a small bowl, combine vinegar, tomato juice and Italian dressing mix. Mix well. Chill.

Lean Lasagna

Low-fat cheese is all that's required to keep the fat content down in this dish.

Yields: 6 3-inch squares
Serving size: 1 3-inch square
Calories per serving: 275

- ½ pound tofu, cubed
- ¼ teaspoon garlic powder
- ½ onion, chopped
- ½ teaspoon dried basil
- 1 6-ounce can tomato paste
- 2 cups water
- ¼ pound lasagna noodles
- 1 cup low-fat cottage cheese
- ¾ pound part-skim mozzarella cheese, sliced
- ½ pound low-fat Cheddar cheese, sliced

To make the sauce, combine tofu, garlic powder, onions, basil, tomato paste and water in a large saucepan. Cover and simmer about 1 hour, stirring occasionally.

Meanwhile, cook noodles according to package directions. Drain and rinse under cold water. Spread out flat until ready to use.

Spray a 6 × 9-inch baking dish with nonstick spray. Spread one-third of the sauce on the bottom of the pan. Top with one-half of the lasagna noodles. Spread cottage cheese over noodles and cover with mozzarella and one-third of the tomato sauce. Top with remaining lasagna, then Cheddar cheese. Pour the rest of the sauce on top.

Bake uncovered in preheated 350°F oven for 45 minutes or until bubbly. Let stand for 10 minutes and then cut into 6 3-inch squares.

Low-Fat Spinach Bake

Yields: approximately 4 cups
Serving size: 1 cup
Calories per serving: 166

- 2 pounds spinach, lightly steamed and drained
- ½ cup chopped onions
- 1 clove garlic, crushed
- ¼ cup low-fat liquid egg substitute
- ¼ cup skim milk
- 2 cups dry-curd cottage cheese
  Dash of freshly ground black pepper
  Dash of nutmeg

Combine spinach, onions, garlic, egg substitute, skim milk and cottage cheese in a 2-quart casserole sprayed with nonstick spray. Sprinkle with pepper and nutmeg. Bake in a preheated 350°F oven for 30 minutes, or until brown and bubbly.

Marinated Halibut

Serves: 2
Calories per serving: 144

- 6 ounces halibut fillets or steaks
- ½ teaspoon salt
- ¼ teaspoon paprika
- ¼ cup chopped onions
- 1½ tablespoons lemon juice

Place halibut in a shallow pan or bowl. Sprinkle with salt, paprika, onions and lemon juice. Cover; let stand 1 hour, turning after 30 minutes. Drain and reserve liquid.

Broil fish in a broiler pan sprayed with nonstick spray 4 inches from heat for 5 minutes on each side, basting with reserved liquid. Serve hot.

Marinated Vegetables

A low-calorie snack you can keep in your refrigerator.

Yields: 2-3 cups
Serving size: ½ cup
Calories per serving: 23

  ½ cup tomato juice
  ¼ cup rice vinegar
  ¼ cup minced celery
  1 tablespoon minced onions
  ¼ teaspoon dried basil
  ¼ teaspoon dried thyme
  1 clove garlic, minced
    Dash of dried tarragon
  ½ cup cauliflowerets
  ½ cup broccoli flowerets
  ½ cup julienned carrots

In a medium-size bowl, combine tomato juice, vinegar, celery, onions, basil, thyme, garlic and tarragon. Set aside.

Blanch cauliflower, broccoli and carrots by placing them in a colander and slowly pouring a large pot of boiling water over them. Pat vegetables dry and place in a medium-size bowl.

Pour the tomato juice mixture over the vegetables, which may be served warm or refrigerated and served cold.

Mashed Squash

Yields: approximately 2 cups
Serving size: ½ cup
Calories per serving: 61

  1 medium acorn squash, halved and seeded
  1 tablespoon maple syrup

  ½ teaspoon pumpkin pie spice
    Butter-flavored salt to taste
    Pepper to taste

Place squash halves cut sides down on a baking sheet sprayed with nonstick spray. Bake in a preheated 400°F oven for 30 minutes, or until tender.

Scoop out squash into a medium-size bowl and beat with an electric mixer. Stir in syrup, pumpkin pie spice, salt and pepper. Serve immediately.

Mollen Milkshake

Filling, nutritious and delicious. A whole meal in one!

Serves: 1
Calories per serving: 350

  1 medium banana, sliced
  1 cup orange juice
  1 cup skim milk
  1 cup strawberries
  1 cup crushed ice

Process all ingredients in a blender until frothy.

Mollen Muffins

Make the dozen and freeze. Defrost one by one as needed.

Yields: 1 dozen
Serving size: 1 muffin
Calories per serving: 103

1½ cups All-Bran cereal
1 cup skim milk
1 egg white
⅓ cup molasses
¼ cup margarine, melted
½ cup all-purpose unbleached white
    flour
½ cup whole wheat flour
2 tablespoons toasted wheat germ
2 teaspoons baking powder
½ teaspoon baking soda
½ cup raisins

In a large bowl, combine cereal and milk and let stand for 3 minutes. Stir in egg white, molasses and margarine. Set aside.

Combine flours, wheat germ, baking powder and baking soda in a large bowl. Make a well in the center. Add bran mixture and stir just until moistened. Fold in raisins. Line a 12-cup muffin tin with paper baking cups; fill two-thirds full.

Bake in a preheated 400°F oven for 20 to 25 minutes. Cool.

Mollenized Sour Cream

A great topping—without the high fat content of real sour cream.

Yields: approximately 1¼ cups
Serving size: 1 tablespoon
Calories per serving: 12

¼ cup skim milk
1 cup low-fat cottage cheese
2 tablespoons lemon juice

Optional ingredients:
¼ cup minced fresh chives
2 tablespoons minced onions
2 tablespoons minced fresh parsley
1 tablespoon Worcestershire sauce

In a small bowl, combine skim milk, cottage cheese and lemon juice. Add optional ingredients (one or more) according to individual taste.

NOTE: This can only be used as a topping. Do not use in cooking.

Mollen's Mushroom Omelet

Serves: 1
Calories per serving: 97

1 medium egg
1 egg white
1 tablespoon water
    Dash of freshly ground pepper
½ cup sliced fresh mushrooms
¼ cup chopped fresh parsley

Place egg, egg white, water and pepper in a small bowl and beat lightly. Stir in the mushrooms and parsley.

Heat an 8- or 9-inch skillet sprayed with nonstick spray. Pour egg mixture into skillet and tilt skillet so that mixture covers the bottom. Cook over low heat until egg is firm, 4 to 5 minutes. Serve immediately.

Mustard Dressing

Yields: 1 cup
Serving size: 1 tablespoon
Calories per serving: 9

1 cup plain, low-fat yogurt
1 tablespoon Dijon mustard
1 tablespoon scallions

In a small bowl, combine all ingredients until well blended. Chill.

Orange-Carrot Salad

Nice and sweet! A nice change from a green salad.

Yields: approximately 3 cups
Serving size: ½ cup
Calories per serving: 49

> 1 tablespoon (1 envelope) unflavored gelatin
> ½ cup orange juice
> 1½ cups boiling water
> ¼ cup lemon juice
> 2 tablespoons sugar
> 3 drops yellow food coloring (optional)
> 1 medium navel orange, peeled and chopped
> ½ cup (1 medium) grated carrots lettuce leaves

In a large bowl, soften gelatin in orange juice. Add boiling water and stir to dissolve gelatin. Stir in lemon juice, sugar and food coloring, if desired. Chill until thickened but not set.

Stir in oranges and carrots. Pour into a 3- to 4-cup mold. Chill 2 to 3 hours until set.

Unmold and serve on lettuce leaves.

Orangey Carrots

Yields: approximately 3 cups
Serving size: ½ cup
Calories per serving: 37

> 3 cups (6 medium) carrots, cut into 2-inch pieces
> ¼ teaspoon paprika
> ½ cup orange juice
> 2 tablespoons chopped onions

In a 1½- to 2-quart casserole or baking dish sprayed with nonstick spray, combine carrots, paprika, orange juice and onions. Stir to mix well.

Bake, covered, in a preheated 350°F oven for 1 hour, or until tender.

Oriental Chicken

Serves: 4
Calories per serving: 205

> 1 fryer chicken (about 1½ pounds), quartered, skin and fat removed
> 1 8-ounce can juice-packed pineapple chunks, drained, juice reserved
> 1½ tablespoons wine vinegar
> 1 tablespoon soy sauce
> ½ teaspoon prepared mustard
> ½ sweet red pepper, julienned
> ½ green pepper, julienned
> 1 teaspoon cornstarch or arrowroot
> 2 tablespoons water

In a large skillet sprayed with non-stick spray, brown chicken pieces, 5 to 10 minutes. Remove and blot.

Place chicken in a shallow baking dish sprayed with nonstick spray. Surround chicken with pineapple chunks.

In a small bowl, combine reserved pineapple juice with vinegar, soy sauce and mustard. Pour over chicken.

Bake, uncovered, in a preheated 350°F oven, basting occasionally, for 30 minutes. Add peppers.

In a cup, stir cornstarch into water and blend well. Stir into liquid in baking dish. Bake 15 minutes more, or until liquid is thick and bubbly.

Parslied Potatoes

Yields: approximately 2 cups
Serving size: ½ cup
Calories per serving: 66

    4 cups water
    2 cups (about 2 medium) peeled,
        quartered red potatoes
    ½ cup chopped fresh parsley

In a large saucepan, bring water to a boil. Add potatoes. Cook, covered, over medium heat for 15 to 20 minutes, or until tender.

Drain potatoes. Add parsley and stir lightly to coat potatoes. Serve hot.

Patio Potato Salad

Potato salad gets its bad reputation as a fattening food because most recipes call for gobs of real mayonnaise, which is 98% fat. Simply by using low-fat mayonnaise and using it sparingly, you can make potato salad part of your low-fat way of life.

Yields: 3-4 cups
Serving size: ½ cup
Calories per serving: 103

    5 cups water
    3 medium potatoes, peeled and cubed
    1½ tablespoons lemon juice
    1 onion, chopped
    3 hard-cooked eggs, quartered
    ½ green pepper, chopped
        Pepper to taste (optional)
    3 tablespoons low-fat mayonnaise

In a large saucepan, bring water to a boil. Add potatoes. Cook, covered, over medium heat for 10 to 15 minutes, or until tender.

Combine potatoes, lemon juice, onions, eggs, green peppers and pepper, if desired, in a large bowl. Toss. Gently stir in mayonnaise, coating potatoes well. Cover and chill.

Pears in Wine

Yields: 2 cups
Serving size: ½ cup
Calories per serving: 90

    2 cups (16-ounce can) juice-packed
        pear halves, drained
    ¼ cup red wine
    1 tablespoon grated lemon peel
    ½ teaspoon cinnamon

In an 8 × 8-inch baking dish or 1-quart casserole, combine all ingredients; mix well.

Bake, uncovered, in a preheated 350°F oven for 15 minutes until hot and bubbly. Serve hot or chill to serve cold.

Pineapple Baked Apple

Yields: 2 apples
Serving size: 1 apple
Calories per serving: 160

    2 large baking apples
    1 8-ounce can juice-packed crushed
        pineapple, drained (juice reserved)
    Water

Core apples without cutting all the way through to the bottom. Peel one-third of way down. Place in a small baking dish. Fill apple centers with pineapple. Add enough water to reserved juice to make ½ cup. Pour liquid into baking dish.

Bake in a preheated 375°F oven for about 1 hour, or until apples are tender. Baste apples with liquid from dish periodically.

Pineapple Pop

You can make just one pop and save the rest of the pineapple for the other dishes that call for pineapple on the 30-day menu plan.

Yields: 8 pops
Serving size: 1 pop
Calories per serving: 90

  1 fresh pineapple
  ½ cup toasted wheat germ

Peel and core pineapple. Cut into 8 wedges and insert a wooden stick into the end of each. Roll in wheat germ (about 1 tablespoon per pop). Stand pops in a jar and freeze.

Poached Chicken Breast

Serves: 2
Calories per serving: 150

  ¼ cup water
  ¼ cup white vinegar
  1 tablespoon lemon juice
  1 teaspoon lemon pepper
  2 teaspoons minced fresh parsley
  1 whole chicken breast, halved, skin and fat removed

In a large skillet, combine water, vinegar, lemon juice, lemon pepper and parsley. Bring to a boil, add chicken, cover and simmer for 20 minutes. Serve hot.

Red Snapper

If you can't find red snapper, substitute another fish, like sole or cod.

Serves: 2
Calories per serving: 113

  ½ pound red snapper fillets, skinned
  ¼ teaspoon dried tarragon
  ¼ teaspoon pepper

  ½ tablespoon minced fresh chives
3 to 4 slices lime

Spray an 8 × 8-inch baking dish with nonstick spray. Arrange fillets in a single layer. Combine tarragon, pepper and chives in a small bowl and sprinkle on top of fish.

Bake in a preheated 375°F oven for 15 to 20 minutes, or until fish flakes when tested with a fork. Garnish with lime slices.

Rice Pilaf

I love rice! Brown rice is high in fiber and a full-cup serving is a lot of eating.

Yields: 1 cup
Serving size: 1 cup
Calories per serving: 247

  1 cup hot cooked brown rice
  2 tablespoons minced onions
  1 teaspoon garlic powder
  1 teaspoon dried mint
  1 teaspoon lemon juice
  1 tablespoon chopped fresh parsley
  Freshly ground pepper to taste

While rice is still steaming hot, gently fold in the onions, garlic powder, mint, lemon juice, parsley and pepper. Serve immediately.

Saucy Chicken and Cheese

A nice use of leftover chicken.

Serves: 1
Calories per serving: 190

    ½ of a 6-ounce jar artichoke hearts,
        drained
    1 teaspoon cornstarch
    ¼ teaspoon instant chicken bouillon
        granules
      Dash of pepper
    ¼ cup skim milk
    ½ cup cubed cooked chicken
    1 tablespoon grated Parmesan cheese
      Dash of paprika
      Minced fresh parsley

Halve any large artichoke hearts. Place artichoke hearts in a small colander and rinse with hot water; drain well. Set aside.

In a medium-size saucepan, combine cornstarch, bouillon granules and pepper. Add skim milk. Cook and stir over medium heat until mixture is thickened and bubbly.

Stir in chicken and artichoke hearts. Transfer chicken mixture to a small (individual) casserole sprayed with nonstick spray. Sprinkle with Parmesan cheese and paprika.

Bake, uncovered, in a preheated 350°F oven for 10 minutes, or until chicken mixture is heated through. Sprinkle with parsley and serve.

Sole and Broccoli with Rice

Sole and broccoli—both low in fat and low in calories.

Serves: 2
Calories per serving: 268

    ½ cup water
    ¼ cup sliced celery

    ½ small onion, sliced
    ½ teaspoon instant chicken bouillon
        granules
    ¼ teaspoon dried tarragon
    ½ pound sole fillets, cubed
    2 ounces Neufchatel cheese, cubed
    1 teaspoon cornstarch
    1 teaspoon cold water
    1 cup hot blanched broccoli flowerets
    1 cup hot cooked brown rice

In a 10-inch skillet, combine water, celery, onions, bouillon granules and tarragon. Bring to a boil. Reduce heat and simmer, covered, for 5 minutes. Add fish; simmer, covered, for 10 to 12 minutes, or until fish flakes easily when tested with a fork. Remove fish with a slotted spoon and keep warm.

Add cheese cubes to cooking liquid. Cook and stir until cheese melts.

In a cup, combine cornstarch and the 1 teaspoon cold water. Add to skillet; cook and stir for 1 minute more. Return fish to sauce; heat through.

To serve, arrange broccoli on hot rice. Top with fish. Pour sauce over fish.

Sole Florentine

Serves: 4
Calories per serving: 130

    ¼ cup minced onions
    ½ teaspoon grated lemon peel
    ½ teaspoon pepper
    ½ teaspoon dry mustard
    2 cups lightly steamed shredded
        spinach, drained
    1 pound sole fillets
    2 tablespoons grated Parmesan cheese
    1 tablespoon minced fresh parsley
    ½ teaspoon paprika

In a skillet sprayed with nonstick spray, combine onions, lemon peel, pepper and mustard and cook over medium heat, stirring frequently, for about 5 minutes. Add spinach and heat through.

Place spinach mixture in an 8 × 8-inch baking dish sprayed with nonstick spray. Place sole on spinach. In a small bowl, combine Parmesan cheese, parsley and paprika and sprinkle on top.

Cover and bake in a preheated 375°F oven for about 15 minutes, or until fish flakes easily when tested with a fork.

Sole with Yogurt Sauce

Serves: 2
Calories per serving: 124

6 ounces sole fillets
½ cup plain, low-fat yogurt
1 tablespoon whole wheat flour
1 tablespoon grated lemon peel
¼ cup minced onions
Dash of paprika
Dash of freshly ground pepper

Place fish in a shallow baking dish sprayed with nonstick spray. In a small bowl, blend yogurt, flour, lemon peel and onions. Pour mixture over fish and sprinkle with paprika and pepper.

Bake in a preheated 350°F oven for 20 to 30 minutes, or until fish flakes easily when tested with a fork.

Sparkling Juice

A wonderful refresher—especially after exercise. Enjoy!

Serves: 1
Calories per serving: 40-90

½ cup club soda
½ cup unsweetened fruit juice

In a small bowl, mix club soda with your choice of fruit juice. Pour over crushed ice in a tall glass and serve immediately.

Spicy Lemon Iced Tea

If you like iced tea, you'll especially enjoy this version.

Yields: 5 cups
Serving size: 1 cup
Calories per serving: 64

4 cups boiling water
5 or 6 decaffeinated tea bags
½ cup lemon juice
¼ cup orange juice
⅓ cup sugar
⅛ teaspoon mint extract, if desired
6 whole cloves
1 cinnamon stick
ice cubes

In a large bowl or 3-quart pitcher, pour boiling water over tea bags. Let steep for 2 to 3 minutes. Remove tea bags. Add remaining ingredients except ice cubes; mix well. Let stand for 5 minutes. Add ice cubes; let stand until chilled before serving.

Spinach Casserole

Yields: approximately 2 cups
Serving size: 1 cup
Calories per serving: 203

1 pound spinach, lightly steamed and drained
¼ cup chopped onions
1 clove garlic, crushed
1 medium egg, beaten
1 cup low-fat cottage cheese
Dash of freshly ground black pepper
Dash of nutmeg

Combine spinach, onions, garlic, egg and cottage cheese in a 2-quart casserole sprayed with nonstick spray. Sprinkle with pepper and nutmeg.

Bake in a preheated 350°F oven for 30 minutes, or until brown and bubbly.

Spinach Royale

Popeye would be jealous!

Yields: 2 cups
Serving size: 1 cup
Calories per serving: 30

  2 cups hot, lightly steamed shredded
     spinach
  1 4-ounce can sliced mushrooms, heated
     in liquid and drained
  2 teaspoons diced onions
    Dash of pepper
    Dash of garlic salt
  1 tablespoon plain, low-fat yogurt

In a large bowl, combine spinach, mushrooms, onions, pepper, garlic salt and yogurt. Toss lightly. Serve immediately.

Stuffed Celery

Wonderful as an appetizer or low-fat snack.

Yields: 12 pieces
Serving size: 1 piece
Calories per serving: 13

  ½ cup low-fat cottage cheese
  1 tablespoon chopped scallions
    Dash of garlic powder
    Dash of cream-style horseradish
    Dash of Worcestershire sauce
  4 large stalks celery, cut into 3-inch
     pieces
    Dash of paprika

In a small bowl, combine cottage cheese, scallions, garlic powder, horseradish and Worcestershire sauce and mix well. Spoon 1 tablespoon cheese mixture into each celery piece. Sprinkle with paprika.

Keep cold in refrigerator until ready to serve.

Stuffed Mushrooms

A nice hors d'oeuvre or accompaniment to a meal.

Yields: 18 mushrooms
Serving size: 1 mushroom
Calories per serving: 11

  18 medium whole fresh mushrooms
  ⅓ cup low-fat cottage cheese
  1 tablespoon chopped fresh chives
    Dash of pepper
  ½ teaspoon Worcestershire sauce
    Dash of paprika

Remove stems from mushrooms and hollow out part of centers, leaving caps intact.

In a small bowl, combine cottage cheese, chives, pepper and Worcestershire sauce. Place 1 tablespoon cheese mixture in each mushroom cap.

Place filled mushrooms, cap side down, on broiler pan or baking sheet sprayed with nonstick spray. Broil 4 to 5 inches from heat for 5 to 7 minutes, or until cheese is melted and mushrooms are slightly brown. Sprinkle with paprika.

Stuffed Potatoes

Potatoes? Fattening? No way! Only 1 percent of the calories in a potato comes from fat.

Yields: 2 potatoes
Serving size: 1 potato half
Calories per serving: 70

  2 medium potatoes
  ¼ cup plain, low-fat yogurt
  2 tablespoons minced fresh chives
  1 tablespoon skim milk
    Dash of garlic powder
    Dash of pepper
  2 tablespoons grated Parmesan cheese
    Paprika

Scrub potatoes; prick with a fork. Bake in a preheated 375°F oven for 60 minutes, or until done. (Leave oven on.)

Slice baked potatoes in half lengthwise. Scoop out pulp, leaving shells intact. Mash potatoes. Add yogurt, chives, milk, garlic powder and pepper. Beat until fluffy. Spoon or pipe potato mixture into potato shells. Sprinkle tops with cheese and paprika.

Return to oven; bake for 10 minutes, or until heated through. If desired, place under broiler to lightly brown tops.

Stuffed Tomato Salad

Take advantage of summer tomatoes for this delightful, easy-to-prepare dish.

Serves: 1
Calories per serving: 128

　1　large tomato
　2　tablespoons chopped fresh chives
　½　cup low-fat cottage cheese
　1　olive

Wedge tomato but do not cut through. (Tomato should look like a flower.)

In a small bowl, mix chives into cottage cheese. Place cottage cheese in the center of the tomato and top with olive.

Tangy Cauliflower

Yields: approximately 2 cups
Serving size: ½ cup
Calories per serving: 27

　2　cups water
　½　teaspoon salt
　1　head cauliflower, divided into flowerets
　½　cup plain, low-fat yogurt
　1　tablespoon minced onions
1 to 2　teaspoons prepared mustard
　½　teaspoon Worcestershire sauce
　　Fresh parsley

In a large saucepan, bring water and salt to a boil; add cauliflower. Cover saucepan and reduce heat; simmer for 8 to 10 minutes, or until tender. Drain.

In a small bowl, combine yogurt, onions, mustard and Worcestershire sauce; mix well. Spread yogurt mixture over cauliflower. Cover; allow to stand until cauliflower has warmed the sauce. Sprinkle with parsley. Serve hot.

Tangy Chicken Salad

Yields: approximately 4 cups
Serving size: ¾ cup
Calories per serving: 230

　½　cup plain, low-fat yogurt
　¼　cup low-fat mayonnaise
　¼　teaspoon curry powder
　1　tablespoon skim milk
　2½　cups diced cooked white-meat chicken
　1　cup sliced celery
　2　tablespoons chopped onions
　½　cup slivered almonds
　　Crisp lettuce leaves

In a large bowl, combine yogurt, mayonnaise, curry powder and milk. Add chicken, celery and onions. Toss well. Chill thoroughly.

Just before serving, mix in almonds. Serve on lettuce leaves.

Tart and Creamy Coleslaw

Yields: 3 cups
Serving size: ½ cup
Calories per serving: 24

  3 cups (about 1 small head) shredded
       or thinly sliced cabbage
  2 tablespoons chopped onions
  1 tablespoon sugar
  2 tablespoons plain, low-fat yogurt
  1 teaspoon lemon juice

In large bowl, combine all ingredients; toss lightly. Chill.

Triple Bean Salad

Beans are a great protein food.

Yields: 3 cups
Serving size: ½ cup
Calories per serving: 61

  1 cup steamed French-style green
       beans
  1 cup steamed yellow wax beans
  1 cup cooked red kidney beans
  1 small onion, thinly sliced
  ¼ cup chopped green peppers
  ¼ cup sugar
  ½ teaspoon pepper
  ¾ cup cider vinegar
  1 tablespoon soy sauce

In a large bowl, combine all ingredients. Cover and chill overnight.

Just before serving, drain well. Toss lightly.

Turkey Chili

Yields: 4-5 cups
Serving size: 1 cup
Calories per serving: 155

  1 cup chopped onions
  3 tablespoons chicken stock
  ½ cup chopped green peppers
  ½ cup chopped sweet red peppers
  1 pound lean ground turkey
  1 16-ounce can chopped tomatoes,
       undrained
  1 teaspoon chili powder
  ½ teaspoon black pepper
       Dash of cayenne

In a large saucepan, sauté onions in stock for 3 minutes, or until they are translucent. Add green peppers and red peppers and simmer for 1 minute more. Add turkey.

When turkey begins to change color (about 5 minutes), add tomatoes, chili powder and black pepper. Bring to a boil and simmer for 15 minutes. Add cayenne and serve.

Turkey-Squash Bake

Serves: 4

Calories per serving: 230

- 2 eggs, lightly beaten
- 1 cup finely crushed saltine crackers
- 1 small scallion, sliced
- ½ teaspoon dried sage
- 2 tablespoons water
- 1 pound lean ground turkey
- 1 12-ounce package frozen mashed cooked winter squash, thawed
- ½ green pepper, sliced
- 1 tablespoon brown sugar
- 1 10-ounce package frozen French-style green beans, cooked according to package directions

In a large bowl, combine 1 egg, half of the crackers, scallions, sage and water and mix. Add turkey and mix again until well blended.

In medium-size bowl, combine squash, remaining crackers, remaining egg, green peppers and brown sugar.

Press half of the turkey mixture into a 9-inch-round, 1½-inch-deep baking dish. Spread squash mixture on top. On wax paper, pat remaining turkey mixture into an 8-inch circle. Invert it onto the squash layer. Remove wax paper.

Bake in a preheated 350°F oven for 40 to 45 minutes. Let stand for 10 minutes; cut into wedges. Serve atop green beans.

Vegetable Kabob

Serves: 1

Calories per serving: 125

- ½ cup red wine vinegar
- 1 tablespoon red wine
- ½ cup water
- ¼ teaspoon dried basil
- ¼ teaspoon dried oregano
  Dash of freshly ground pepper
- 1 clove garlic, crushed
- 4 large fresh mushrooms
- 2 slices eggplant, cut into chunks and broiled until soft
- ½ medium onion, cut into chunks
- ½ large pepper, cut in wide strips
- 6 cherry tomatoes

In a large bowl, combine wine vinegar, wine, water, basil, oregano, pepper and garlic and stir. Add mushrooms, eggplant, onions, peppers and tomatoes. Let stand at room temperature for 1 hour.

Drain vegetables, reserving marinade. Alternate vegetables onto a large skewer. Broil 4 inches from heat, turning and basting frequently with reserved marinade, for about 7 minutes.

Waldorf Salad

Yields: 2 cups
Serving size: ½ cup
Calories per serving: 110

  1½ cups diced apples
  ½ teaspoon lemon juice
  2 medium celery stalks, sliced
  ¼ cup broken walnuts
  1 tablespoon sugar
  ¼ cup plain, low-fat yogurt
  1 tablespoon low-fat mayonnaise
    Crisp lettuce leaves

Place apples in a medium-size bowl and drizzle lemon juice over them; toss well. Mix in celery and walnuts.

In a small bowl, blend together sugar, yogurt and mayonnaise. Fold into apple mixture. Chill.

Serve on lettuce leaves.

Whole Wheat Bran Pancakes

Yields: 4 cakes
Serving size: 2 cakes
Calories per serving: 138

  1½ cups skim milk
  1 egg white
  ½ cup all-purpose unbleached white
    flour
  ½ cup whole wheat flour
  ¼ cup wheat bran
  2 tablespoons safflower or corn oil
  1¼ teaspoons baking powder

In a large bowl, combine milk, egg white, flours, bran, oil and baking powder and mix until batter is fairly smooth.

For each pancake, pour ¼ cup batter onto a *lightly* oiled griddle heated to 400°F. Turn pancakes when tops are covered with bubbles and edges look browned. Brown lightly and serve.